LIVING MEDICINE

LIVING MEDICINE

Memoir Snapshots

V. L. BECKETT, MD

To order additional copies of this book, contact:
Xlibris Corporation
1-888-795-4274
www.Xlibris.com
Orders@Xlibris.com
25910

CONTENTS

This book is dedicated to my father and mother,
and my husbands, Peter and Joe,
for their unstinting love and support.

INTRODUCTION &

ACKNOWLEDGEMENTS

In the telling of my life events, I hope to convey my gratitude to America, my adopted country, for the opportunities she has given me. My diverse experiences cover laughter and tears in China, Ireland, Cuba and the U.S.

I have been privileged to take part in the brightest field of human endeavor—medicine, and to work in the finest medical institution I have ever known—the Mayo Clinic. My description of how this institution works may interest people at large but especially patients and would-be patients.

As I have grown older, I have come to grips with resolving past problems, and to plan a future that addresses physical, mental, emotional and spiritual life aspects. I have found some answers that may help others in their searches.

For their privacy, I have not used real names of significant persons who are still living. I have relied on memory (which can be wrong), written reports of my father, information gleaned from newspapers and public articles on Mayo, travel guides and, of course, my references, but any errors are entirely mine. This book reflects my individual views and opinions, and does not necessarily reflect those of the Mayo Clinic, or other institutions herein mentioned. All Mayo photos are by permission of Mayo Foundation for Medical Education and Research.

I wish to thank my medical mentors and patients for the lessons they taught me, and my family, friends and colleagues for their helpful advice. Special thanks to reviewers of the manuscript in its various revisions: Claire Van Zant, an eminent English teacher, Dr. Linda Butterfield, ophthalmologist friend and Kathleen Stoehr, my professional editor. Their suggestions have greatly improved the book. My gratitude extends to my Xlibris editors, and especially, to my husband Joe, who walked every step with me to bring this book to fruition.

MAJOR CHINA DYNASTIES

Qin dynasty   (221–207 BCE)

Han dynasty   (c. 200 BCE–200 CE)

Multiple Kingdoms   (c. 200–600 CE)

Tang dynasty   (c. 600–900 CE)

Song dynasty   (c. 900–1300 CE)

Yuan dynasty (Mongols)   (c. 1300–1400 CE)

Ming dynasty   (1368–1644)

Qing dynasty (Manchus)   (1644–1911)

Republic of China

(Nationalist Government)   (1912–1949)

People's Republic of China

(Communist Government)   (1949–present)

(c. = circa; CE = Common Era, previously called AD;
BCE = previously called BC)

Chapter 1

THE LAST SCHOLAR

Ling Ping, my father, was living in a Chinese village in Henan Province in the year 1905 of the Qing Dynasty. The noonday sun of the eighth month was hot on his young brown body, which was shielded only by a pair of old, blue cotton pants. Deep in thought, he lay on top of the water buffalo he was tending. How could he persuade his father to let him take the imperial examination in the prefecture[1] capital? These civil service examinations were open to all, but there could be a fuss. After all, he was only twelve years old. With a laugh he thought, I'll tell Father that my passing the examination will bring honor and glory to our village and family. He could not object to that. I'm sure I can pass. Didn't my tutor say I was the brightest student in the whole countryside?

Decision made, he patted his pigtail braided with red string, then jabbed his heels into the water buffalo's side, driving him toward his village. He left the animal in its shed and ran down a short lane to arrive breathless at his brick home. Barging into a small room on the side of the courtyard, he found his tutor, book in hand, teetering back and forth in his chair as he read in

---

[1]   Prefecture: geographical unit of government, several of which make up a province.

a soft singsong. A small thin man with a wispy beard, he wore a black skull cap, a long black cotton gown, and displayed the two-inch long curling fourth and fifth fingernails, typical of a scholar who did no manual work.

Peering over his book, he said, "Ah, Xiao Ping (Little Ping), what are you up to?"

After a quick bow, Ping poured out his ideas.

The tutor nodded. "I think it can be done." They laid plans to speak with Ping's father after supper.

Supper was an hour before sundown, around the sixth hour. As usual, his father discussed the crops and the tutor answered in monosyllables, while Ping, his mother, and nine brothers and sisters silently ate their rice, chicken and vegetables. After supper the others retired, leaving the two men to talk. His tutor motioned Ping to stay.

"Landlord Ling," he said, "your son has a request."

Ping looked at the two men he most admired and respected. How different they were. His tutor was profound and knowledgeable in literature and philosophy, but wholly impractical. Conversely, his father was forceful and practical, a man who had elevated himself from a tenant farmer to a small landowner. A tall Northerner with a strong, muscular build, he wore the blue cotton jacket and pants of a farmer. At forty-one, his clean-shaven face was unlined and his piercing eyes missed little.

Ping, the ninth of ten children, knew he was his father's favorite. Since age four, he had studied with this outstanding private tutor, and his quick mind and retentive memory delighted both men. By twelve, he was thoroughly grounded in the Four Books and Five Classics of Confucius philosophy. His calligraphy[2] was good, and he could compose passable poetry—

---

[2]   Calligraphy: brush writing of Chinese characters.

all requirements for the examinations. But was this enough to convince his father?

"Well," said his father, impatiently.

"Father, I would like your permission to take the imperial examinations at the prefecture capital in one month's time," he blurted.

There was a long silence.

His father turned to the tutor. "Is he ready?"

The tutor nodded, "Yes. Landlord Ling, he is as ready as any pupil I have ever had. I believe this boy will do extraordinary things; he has a bright future. After all, your wife's Fong family has many famous scholars, so scholarship is not new to your family. This examination is only the first and lowest of four levels of examinations[3]. When he passes, he will earn an imperial post. What a fine distinction for our village."

"But he is so young to journey to the capital."

"No need to worry, sir. His older cousins and elder brother already plan to take the examination. Ping can join them." He added with a twinkle in his eye, "The cousin who is repeating the examination knows the procedure well."

Both men laughed, and Ping sighed with relief. But before his cautious father would give approval, he consulted a fortune-

---

[3]   Competitive imperial exams: (c.600 CE-1906) Chinese system of selecting scholars of high standing for government administrative posts, thereby giving young men, even from remote rural areas, access to government posts. There were four degrees: First, shu-cheh, equivalent to western BA degree, Second, equivalent to MA degree, Third, equivalent to Ph.D. degree, Fourth, highest degree given personally by the emperor. Each degree recipient could obtain a government post, the lower posts to the lower level degree winners, the highest to Fourth degree winners.

teller—a procedure before weighty decisions. The fortune-teller said Ping would definitely be a winning candidate.

Returning to the tutor, his father said, "So be it. I will hire a man to carry him in a wheelbarrow when he tires of walking. Please calculate how much money he will need. I will inform his companions." Smiling at Ping, he patted his small head. "As for you, young man, study hard, do your best and enjoy your great adventure."

Ping was so excited, he hardly noticed the physical demands of the week long journey. Fortunately, his cousins took care of everything. A strong young boy, Ping walked most of the way himself.

They arrived at the capital three days before the examination started. For two days Ping wandered the streets of the capital, clinging to his cousin's hand, eyes wide with wonder. Soldiers and noblemen in brightly colored silk clothes rode horses whose shoes clattered against the large flat stones of the streets. Teams of four men hoisted sedan chairs to transport beautiful young women. Sedate men and women of all ages rode around in *rickshaws*[4]. Among the crowds, many farmers pushed carts piled high with vegetables or fruits. Ping had never seen so many people, nor heard such a din of talking, shouting and hawking of wares. When the smell of food being cooked in the street stalls made Ping hungry, his cousin treated him to a bowl of chicken noodle soup topped with vegetables, and a steamed bun stuffed with dates.

In a residential area, he saw walled single-story houses built five feet from the street. Their barely visible red-tiled roofs

---

[4]   Rickshaw: a small two-wheeled carriage with a hood, pulled by one man.

had up-tilting corners, which his cousin explained were to keep evil spirits from stopping. In the commercial section, shops lined the streets. Ping especially enjoyed buying a small blue bowl for his mother, silk handkerchiefs for his sisters and books for his father and brothers. Tired and happy, they returned to sleep at the inn, which was already filling with other candidates and their families.

On examination morning they were wakened at the fourth hour by the deafening roar of a single cannon shot. Rapidly dressing and breakfasting, Ping and his companions were ready to leave at the second cannon volley an hour later. Each candidate carried a basket containing an inkstone, a black ink stick, brush-pens, lunch and water. When they arrived at the outer gate of the huge examination hall, they looked for others from their district.

Ping had been told that this prefecture was composed of five districts, each sending about a thousand candidates to compete for the thirty-five degrees to be conferred. His cousin pointed out the district magistrates, district school staff and their students, also called local licentiates. At the third cannon shot, the great doors opened. Ping was separated from his companions as he was swept through the door to line up at the second gate. After the prefecture clerks thoroughly searched them for books, notes or other suspicious objects that might be used for cheating, Ping and the others entered the examination hall in groups of twenty. Each candidate bowed to the Prefect as they passed in front of him.

The huge hall became very quiet as the candidates waited at their desks. Ping sat at a desk near the front, so could not see his companions. The Imperial Chief Examiner entered and took his seat on a raised platform in the center of the hall. Ping looked with awe at a man who was at least two heads taller than his father and twice his girth. He wore a long magenta gown of silk tapestry, and a flat ceremonial black hat that jutted out in front and at both sides. His alert eyes in a smooth, round face gazed calmly at the roomful of candidates.

As each name was called, the candidate came forward and bowed to this official. Ping followed suit. After a local licentiate, acting as guarantor, confirmed his identity as a candidate, Ping was allowed to pick up a set of examination papers and return to his seat. These papers were in the form of a folded book of plain white paper with red ruled vertical lines. On the corner of the cover, a small label was stamped with three seals. As instructed, Ping wrote his name on the label, tore it off and kept it together with his seat number in his pocket. He then wrote his name and seat number on top of the examination paper. Since his name would be covered during grading of his paper, only his seat number identified his answers until the end of the grading. When all the examination papers were distributed, the guarantors, teachers and magistrates left the hall, and the Chief Examiner locked and sealed the gate behind them. The examination promptly started. Ping stole a look at the candidates next to him and stifled a laugh at their serious mien.

The examination questions were written on lighted lanterns that were carried around the hall by stewards. They were selected passages from the Confucian classical books. The candidate was to write an essay on them, quote a commentary by a specific famous scholar, and conclude with his own explanation. Ping thought the questions easy. After two hours, another set of questions was paraded about. One was to explain another passage from the Four Books, the other was to compose a poem on a given theme, using five characters to a line and set to a given rhyme. They had the afternoon to complete their work.

The strict monitoring of these examinations had been explained to Ping. Whenever a candidate did something improper, a clerk immediately approached his desk and stamped the appropriate seal on his paper. The ten different seals were:

1. Leaving one's seat (they were allowed only one leave for a drink or to go to the toilet)
2. Exchanging papers
3. Dropping a paper
4. Talking
5. Gazing around and looking at another's papers
6. Changing seats
7. Disobeying (failing to comply with the clerk's instructions)
8. Violating regulations
9. Humming (this happened when candidates composed rhymes for poems—to the great annoyance of others)
10. Not completing the examination (when a paper was not finished at the end of the day, this stamped seal prevented later additions).

One such stamp did not disqualify a candidate, but it could seriously influence the judge's impression. Another cause for failure was illegible calligraphy, so Ping was to write with careful brush strokes.

Ping looked around; he didn't want to miss anything he could later describe to his brothers and young village friends. Finally, he lowered his head to concentrate on the questions, and began to write. He had no trouble remembering the passages or the scholar's commentary, but his own explanation took time. When he needed to use the toilet, he raised his hand. The clerk gave him permission, also allowed him to eat some flat bread and drink some tea. He smiled his approval when Ping returned promptly.

Composing poetry, the next step in the examination, was not his favorite task. Hearing footsteps, he looked up to see the Chief Examiner. Ping immediately stood and bowed.

"Sit down. Sit down. Continue with your work," the man encouraged. After Ping sat, the official looked over his writing, then nodded, smiled and moved away. The boy was so astonished he had trouble concentrating, but finally his mind cleared and he finished the poem.

At the fourth hour of the afternoon, the clerks called out in loud voices, "Quickly submit your papers." Ping checked his answers, made sure he had his name slip with seat number, then handed in his paper and received a bamboo tally, an exit pass, to throw into a basket near the inner gate. Later, he and his companions walked in tired silence to the inn. They slept late the next morning, since the examination results would not be available for a week.

Ping and his companions argued vigorously over the answers to the examination questions. When they pulled out books to check, his brother and two cousins were startled to find their answers wrong. Discouraged, they realized they had probably failed.

To cheer them up, Ping told them of the Chief Examiner's visit to his desk and asked what they thought. They looked alarmed and asked, "Did you do anything improper?" Ping told them of his brief departure from his desk, but assured them no seal had been placed on his examination paper. Everyone was mystified.

The first examination results were released a week later. Tensely the candidates gathered at the outer gate of the examination hall as the names of passing candidates were posted on the gate. Ping was too small to see over the heads of the other candidates, so his cousin lifted him onto his shoulders. Perched there, Ping found his name, the sixteenth of about five hundred candidates from his district who passed. None of his companions' names were posted.

Dejected, Ping's companions could not sleep that night. The next morning they stayed at the inn, while Ping went alone to the examination hall for the second session. The remaining candidates sat in their former seats and again wrote their seat numbers on their examination papers. This session's questions were similar to those of the first. He easily answered the first part, and was beginning the second part when he again heard approaching footsteps.

The Chief Examiner put his hand on Ping's shoulder and whispered to him not to rise. He took out his ink brush and made red circles at the end of several sentences on Ping's paper, each time saying, "*Hao* (Good)." The red circle indicated his approval. As the Examiner walked back to his seat in the center of the hall, Ping felt puzzled. He had never heard of such a thing, but the red approval circles appeared to be a good sign. With renewed energy, he quickly answered the second question, and then composed a short poem. As before, he was in the first group to leave the examination hall. He detoured from his return to the inn to search for interesting sights. After all, he thought, I might not be back here again. He found some entertainers on the streets, including a puppet show that fascinated him, but he soon returned to the inn.

Ping's companions scolded him for going out alone in a strange city. They listened intently to the happenings in the examination hall, and remained mystified at the actions of the Examiner. A few days later, the second test results were announced. This time Ping's name was sixth on the list among the one hundred fifty passing candidates from his district.

The following morning, Ping went for the third and final examination. One question was from the Five Classics. Next, he was to write two essays, one on a historical event and one on government policies. Looking around for a familiar face, he saw the Chief Examiner beckoning him. He instructed a clerk to set Ping's desk and chair next to his on the platform. "Small candidate, please do your work by me," he said. Everyone in the room looked surprised, especially Ping. With the Chief Examiner looking over his shoulder, he was too nervous to write. When finally the Examiner went for a walk, Ping recovered his confidence and wrote a few terse answers. Ping was ready to hand in his paper when the Examiner returned. He took the paper from the boy and led him to a small room off the hall. After both were seated, the Chief Examiner read his answers, and again circled the passages he liked with red ink.

"You write very well, young man. What is your proper name?"

"Ling Ping, sir."

"What is your age?"

"Twelve, sir."

He nodded. "Yes, very young. It has been a long time since one of your age has passed these qualifying tests. Tell me your father's name and where you live. I would like to send him a message." When Ping told him, the official wrote a short message on a piece of paper that he folded, sealed and handed to Ping. "What do you think of staying with me at the provincial capital and letting me supervise your studies?"

"Why, sir, I don't know what to say," he stuttered in confusion.

"Think about it and discuss it with your father. You would progress far faster under my care than in your village."

His companions were thunderstruck when Ping told them what happened. His cousin finally said, "You have made a fine impression; this could be an important opportunity for you. Your father will help you decide."

In the final results, Ping was the first among the thirty-five successful candidates for the first degree. He and his companions danced for joy. Ping was instructed to bring the label with his name and desk number to the prefect for name verification as a winning candidate. Then his cousin took Ping to buy the prescribed clothing of a new *shu-cheh* (recipient of the first level degree), a small black cap and a blue mandarin garment bordered in black. At the banquet honoring the winners, Ping followed the other *shu-cheh* as they bowed and thanked the Chief Examiner and his staff. The official then gave each an ornament of gold foil, known as the "gold flower," which he attached to their caps. He smiled broadly at Ping and reminded him to give his message to his father. Ping bowed in reply.

Ping's group left for home the next morning. Word spread rapidly, and at every stop he was feasted in celebration of his achievement. He felt overwhelmed. A mile from Ping's village, the elders, his family and his tutor came to greet him. He could scarcely believe his eyes when they laid red rugs on the ground for him to walk on. Then he realized that this was their way of thanking him for bringing honor to their village.

After the excitement abated, Ping handed his father the Chief Examiner's message. His father exclaimed in surprise, "He wishes to adopt you as his son and give you a suitable education!" After a pause, he declared, "I cannot allow that. You are my son. I will provide for your education. We can start plans right away."

Historical Note: The following year, 1906, the competitive imperial examination was abolished. Although it had given China's administrative service the brightest minds and had held the huge empire together for thirteen hundred years, its emphasis on ancient classics and philosophical teachings while neglecting modern practical and scientific ways could not continue. Then in 1911, the Qing Dynasty itself fell and gave way to the Republic of China.

Post Script: Throughout my childhood, I heard my father tell and retell this story of his taking the Imperial examinations. After the examinations, the village could no longer hold my father. He went on to attend Nankai High School in the city of Tianjin, port city to Beijing. Later, the government sponsored his study in America, where he obtained his BA from Stanford University and his Ph.D. in psychology from Clark University. Upon returning to China, he helped build the university section of Nankai University, then was active in the government's Foreign Ministry, representing China in many foreign countries. Our family was immensely proud of him. Because of travel difficulties to the isolated rural countryside, he returned to his home village to visit his parents only a few times.

In 1944 he came to the United States to represent China in the Bretton Woods International Monetary Conference. Our family had a happy reunion in New York City. His political career came to an end when the Communists took control of China in 1949. He received various consultant assignments, such as advisor to the Bank of China in New York City, so he elected to stay on in New York with my mother. For several years he taught political science at the local university. His apartment became the center for expatriates to gather and discuss personal and international events. Until his death at age ninety-four, he continued to study Chinese history and ponder China's future; I can still hear him telling stories and repeating quotations from Chinese classics. I believe he was the last of a remarkable class, the Chinese scholar-official–

steeped in Confucius classics and high ethical standards, and devoted to the government and people he served.

He taught me to reach for high goals and to always be honorable. He instilled in me a love of learning that he believed built character and led to a successful, fulfilling life. I was to discover the truth of this for myself.

Chapter 2

TIANJIN: EARLY CHILDHOOD 1923-30

A faded 5x3 black-and-white photograph tugs at my earliest memories. Turning it over, I see the label says I am three years old. I stand between my younger sister and older brother; our bulky, quilted Chinese gowns make us look like plump little sausages with arms. Mother and Aunt stand behind us, wearing fur-collared coats and wool hats. Behind them is our small one-story home, indistinguishable in a row of Nankai University faculty houses. The university is in Tianjin, a North China port city, frigid in winter from bitter north Mongolian winds, but blistering in summer. On the day of the photograph, the air must have been biting and harsh.

My parents and aunt, who also lived with us, all taught at Nankai University. Since Father, the Dean, was usually away on school assignments, he seemed an exotic stranger during his brief returns. When he was home, I would sit on a tiny stool next to his chair and shyly gaze up at him. With a broad smile, he would pat my head, saying, "My little quiet one, how have you been?" Nodding vigorously I would whisper, "Good, Father. Good." During dinner, he enthralled us with stories of his encounters with generals and government officials or painted pictures of colorful provinces he had traveled to, his rich voice rising and falling and his expressive hands gesturing to emphasize his points. Just as we felt complete, happy and whole, he would be gone again.

In his absence, Mother was the bulwark of our family. She quietly hurried back and forth from home to her teaching duties at school. I did not realize then how purposeful she was; to me she was just a rock steady, guiding force in my life. A plump five feet, she combed her hair back in a smooth bun and wore simple, dark-colored Chinese long-gowns. Behind her round-faced gentle smile were a quiet dignity and an aura of strength. Only her sparkling dark eyes hinted of the energy with which she pursued life and her family's welfare. She was, and has always been, my role model.

My brother, sister and I, thirteen months apart in age, each had a personal *amah* (nanny). Mother wanted someone home with us when she was away at the University. Our *amahs* were simple low-paid country women who lived in the servants' quarters, and returned infrequently to their homes. Mother forbade them to spank us, so they made us obey by telling us frightening ghost stories! This suited us fine, since we relished the wonderful folk tales of ancient colorful heroes, satanic black-faced warriors and wicked beautiful sorceresses. Sometimes we would be deliberately naughty, just to hear another tale.

But we did have an occasional frightening threat. Roving bandits regularly passed near our area—part of the revolutionary turmoil engulfing other parts of the country. With Father away, the only adult male at home was our cook, Ah-Wang. Ordinarily mild mannered and friendly, Ah-Wang became fiercely protective when he thought our family was in danger. A tall, wiry ex-army soldier, trained to use the fearsome "Big Sword" (a broad blade about two feet long), he would check the security of doors and windows, and at night sleep on the front doorstep with his weapon strapped to his waist. "Do not be afraid," he told Mother, "I will protect you from harm." We felt safer to see him on guard. Fortunately, no bandits attacked the campus when we were there.

The seasons merged one pleasurable period into another. Our family spent summer holidays at Bei-dai He, a seaside resort north of Tianjin, where we frolicked in the salty waves and spent blissful afternoons building sand castles on the beach. Winters on Nankai campus delighted us with ice skating and ice sledding on nearby frozen ponds and rivers. Play and laughter filled those carefree days.

My religious education was certainly not the norm for a child growing up in China. Most Chinese are Buddhists who follow the philosophy of Confucius and Lao Tzu. My agnostic Father left Mother to teach us religion. My maternal grandfather was one of the early Chinese Presbyterian ministers, so as minister's children, my mother and aunt were solid Presbyterians, welcoming many American missionaries to our home. I remember looking forward to seeing a jolly bearded missionary who brought jars of honey along with a loaf of bread. He would tell stories of Jesus as we nibbled on his treats. Mother wanted us taught Christian beliefs about the love of Jesus, what was right and wrong and compassion for others. The missionaries we knew were cheerful sincere people, seemingly undaunted by the task of teaching Christianity in a land of Buddhists.

Another approach to Christianity came from my aunt's sweet-faced missionary friend, Minta, a piano teacher, who brought Christianity into our lives through music. Sitting nearby I would watch and listen as these two young women talked, laughed and played the piano, wishing with all my heart to grow up as graceful and attractive as they were. I became very fond of "Aunt" Minta. She introduced me to classical Western music, especially to Mozart, Beethoven and Chopin, which even today brings back memories of my Tianjin years.

Sometime during those early seven years, I became aware of two starkly contrasting people who lived outside our family and campus circle. Mother occasionally took me on visits to her wealthy friend in the city. I vividly recall an enormous house, and elaborately carved wooden chairs that I found most uncomfortable to sit on. Bright red peonies filled big, colorful ceramic pots. Although the rooms were beautiful and luxurious I never felt at ease there. However, two courtyard peacocks fascinated me, parading daintily on thin spindly legs and spreading their iridescent blue-green tail feathers into lovely wide-open fans.

Conversely, Mother led us into the small village near our campus, to bring food and clothing to the poor. People here looked tired, wore ragged clothes and lived in small huts with mud floors. In summer the children ran naked. In winter the entire family spent the day and slept the night on a large *kang,* a brick platform warmed underneath by a fire. Mother was thanked profusely for the food and clothing we brought. I wondered why I, without deserving it, had the comfort and security these people couldn't have. I vowed to someday help the poor and unfortunate.

Grandmother Ling's visit caused great excitement. With considerable relief Mother said, "This means she and Grandfather have finally forgiven your father for marrying me." Northern and southern Chinese had long distrusted each other because they spoke different dialects and had different ways. Mother from a southern province, and father from a northern province met while studying in California and later married. Father's parents strongly disapproved of their marriage. Grandfather said, "She is not only a southerner, but educated, so likely to be troublesome." Father refused to listen, so Grandfather cut off further communication. With the passing of years, as Mother proved a wonderful wife and mother, their stance began to soften. Grandmother especially wanted to see her grandchildren, so here she was. Throughout the visit, Mother was a warm and gracious hostess, and Father never seemed to stop smiling.

Grandmother was a tiny figure teetering on small bound feet. Her wrinkled face was wreathed in smiles; her gray-streaked black hair was tightly pulled back into a bun and held by a lovely green jade hairpin; and she wore the common black cotton tunic and trousers of country folk. She had traveled with considerable effort from her village several hundred miles away in Henan province. I realized this could be the only time we would ever see her.

Because of our intense curiosity in her bound feet, one evening she allowed my sister and I to watch her daily feet-washing ritual. When she unwrapped her feet, we saw that her poor forefeet had been deformed by tight wrappings as a child, so she actually walked on her heels. While her feet were no longer painful, walking was difficult because of her poor balance.

"How did this happen?" I asked.

She hesitated, then in a quiet voice explained, "It started in the Qing dynasty, when a high official said he preferred to marry a girl with small feet. It became a fashion craze, and mothers started to bind their little girl's feet to make them small, so that later she would be acceptable for a good marriage." How dreadful, I thought.

Grandmother said, "My mother hated to put me through this painful ordeal, but was afraid not to, afraid she would limit my chances for a proper marriage. I'm so glad for you two girls that the new government has forbidden this practice." Sister and I heartily agreed. Recognizing her difficulty, we fought to hold her hands and steady her whenever she walked. As I began to know her better, I grew to love this indomitable, enterprising little woman.

She took time to show us how she made "thousand year eggs," a type of preserved eggs prized to this day in China. We watched as she sat on a stool in the backyard and made a black paste of ashes and special powders. Then she completely covered a dozen large, fresh duck eggs with this paste, wedged them in a large clay pot and buried the pot in the ground, marking the spot with a wooden label. We were not to touch the pot for at least six months, after which Cook could remove it, take out individual eggs, crack open the shell and serve them as a treat. The eggs would be brown-black, with the consistency and taste of smoky hard-boiled eggs, and to our palate, delicious. This visit was her only one, a delightful experience I never forgot.

But the figure who loomed largest in those years was Mother. She took care of our family's every need, as well as managed the house and servants. Although she taught full time, she read stories to us, often in English, giving us an early start in the language that was to supercede our native Chinese. Somehow, without preaching, she instilled in us our responsibilities and the difference between right and wrong. "It is wrong," she said, "to lie or hurt others. You must be truthful and polite, obey and respect your elders, and be kind to those who work for us." When my brother talked back, she punished him by swatting his legs with a roll of newspapers; she scolded the three of us whenever we fought among ourselves. Because she was fair, we tried hard to behave to avoid distressing her. Another trait was her health consciousness. Our campus neighbors were askance when they heard she washed uncooked salad ingredients with potassium permanganate, bought a goat so we could drink milk, or fed us cod liver oil in orange juice each morning. "Such Western ways," they whispered.

She was also a good teacher, strict but well liked by her students. On many afternoons our house would be filled with excited, cheerful students who came to tea, and often stayed for supper as they talked about school and the problems of the day. The new republic was an engrossing topic of discussion. Zhou Enlai, later to become premier of China, was one of her students. Mother said he was very bright, but seldom studied and often skipped classes because he was just too busy organizing student demonstrations. She was never happier than when the house was full of students. "These are the leaders of the future," she proudly stated. In my pride in my remarkable mother, I imitated her speech and gestures, which made the students laugh.

We three grew and thrived in Tianjin. When I was about seven, however, Father came home one day in great excitement. He had just been appointed the Chinese minister to Cuba, and ambassador-at-large of the Caribbean area. When asked, "Where is Cuba?" Father showed us on the map. "Here, in the Caribbean Sea, near America. It is a tropical island. You will love it there."

As we busily packed, I wondered, would I miss Tianjin? Only in retrospect, did I value this tranquil oasis in my early childhood. Soon I was about to experience a whole new way of life, with new excitement and new dangers.

Chapter 3

HAVANA, CUBA 1930-35

I n 1930 my parents, older brother, younger sister and I left our small house on a university campus in chilly North China, to come to live in a mansion on this Cuban tropical island. Father immediately took up his duties, Mother took care of house and family as well as served as hostess for Father, and we three eagerly acquainted ourselves with our new home and the people in this foreign land.

Initially, I found this transformation hard to believe; new experiences happened quickly. Let me start with a time four years after arrival, when I was beginning to feel settled.

One spring day in 1934, when I was about ten, I stepped out of our black chauffeured limousine in front of an elegant, three-story, cream-colored Spanish style mansion on a fashionable street in Havana. I glanced with satisfaction at a big, shining brass plate on the tall black wrought-iron gate that read:

La Legacion de China en Cuba
(Chinese Legation in Cuba)

My father lived here as the Chinese Minister to Cuba, and as the oldest daughter, I felt like a princess living in a palace.

As I walked through the now familiar iron gate, part of a high protective iron fence that surrounded the house, I entered a small garden where we often played at dusk, when it was cooler. We would scamper noisily amid the stately palms, large bright red and yellow flowers, and strange tropical trees. Inside the mansion, the high ceilings and marble floors kept the house cool when it was scorching outdoors, and we found plenty of rooms to play hide-and-seek. "Mother, I'm home now," I called. "Good," came her voice from within, "change your clothes, and go play with your brother and sister outside before it gets dark."

Our house staff consisted of Anna, the black maid who cleaned, washed, sewed and ironed and told us Cuban folk tales; Ah-ming, the young Chinese houseboy who ran all the errands and played checkers with us; and Ah-ki, the small elderly Chinese cook who kept shooing us out of his basement kitchen. Since they only spoke Spanish, we quickly learned enough of the language to tease them.

We enrolled in the Havana German School, run by German expatriates for children of well-to-do and diplomatic families. Most of the classes were in English, a few in Spanish and German was an elective. Imagine my brother's surprise when he finished a German class to receive a certificate signed by the already controversial Hitler. The classes were easy, so I spent my time making friends; my favorites turned out to be the daughters of the American and Japanese ambassadors, perhaps because we came from similar diplomatic households. However, I found one difficult class—gym. The teacher was a gray-haired, heavy-muscled man of military bearing who shouted, "*Dummkopf* (dumb head)" whenever we did not perform to his exacting standards. On the annual Parent's Day, we students gave an outstanding gymnastic demonstration, but we trembled as we performed under this teacher's baleful gaze that seemed to say, "Don't you dare make a mistake."

In the hot weather, we naturally wanted to swim, but the waters were shark-infested so inviting beaches were forbidden to swimmers. Instead, Father put us in the elite Havana Country Club, where watchful teachers taught us swimming. Even then, one day a shark managed to breach the metal fences that cordoned off the swimming area. Frantic cries of "Sharks! Sharks!" sent everyone scurrying for land. In spite of these risks, I soon enjoyed heavenly times splashing in the warm, sparkling-blue Caribbean waters. We also loved going to the movies. Somehow Mother ferreted out a cinema that put on American children's movies. I remember standing in line to pay 25 *centavos* (cents) to see *Our Gang*. I doubt it improved my English, but it was fun.

Father's work was all-important. After years of seeing him only on rare occasions in China, it was a treat to see him daily. The legation's office rooms took up most of the second floor, our smaller living quarters were behind. I used to stand quietly by the doorway peeking in to watch the activities. After reading the morning newspapers in English, Spanish and Chinese, Father would confer with Wong Chu, the dapper Chinese secretary from China, or with Jose Delgado, the stolid Cuban secretary who spoke English and Spanish. He would then dictate letters to them in English or Chinese, and Delgado then translated various English ones into Spanish. In the afternoon, "Mr. Minister," as everyone called him, had daily appointments to see visitors—Cuban, Chinese and American.

Father was a slender, quick-moving man, with a mobile face, expressive hands and a clear, confident voice. His sharp intelligence did not tolerate fools, but he laughed often and made friends easily. Fiercely patriotic, he proudly represented China in Cuba. Some days, wearing top hat and tuxedo he dropped by government offices; other days, in a light gray suit he visited people around the island.

Although he could be tense and methodical during the working day—even showing flashes of temper—Father was usually relaxed and cheerful in the evening over our simple family meal. At the table he enthralled us with stories of his experiences with Chinese fortune-tellers and trips in Europe, or stories from Chinese history about warrior feats and emperor intrigues. His infectious belly laugh would spark our answering laughter—he enjoyed the telling as much as we enjoyed the listening. In the evenings, he often invited cronies to play poker. Father had an inscrutable poker face; no one could guess what hand he held. When he won, you could hear his laughter all over the house. We always knew where Father was. He was the noisy parent and Mother the quiet one, who ensured things ran smoothly behind the scenes.

My father worked hard to be a good minister, especially to help the Chinese men who originally came to work the Cuban sugar-cane fields, and later rose to become farmers and small store owners. They particularly appreciated his efforts to change a Cuban law so they could bring wives from China, since they preferred Chinese wives. On another occasion, Father insisted on banning a particularly demeaning movie about the Chinese. When the Cuban government ignored his request, Father threatened to leave Cuba unless the government complied. When they called his bluff, he abruptly drove to the airport, ready to leave. Alarmed, the Cuban officials gave in and hurriedly stopped him. One of them laughingly told Mother, "We like and respect him. He is a fighter." Mother later told us in confidence that Father was so sure of the result, he never even bothered to tell her he was going to the airport!

Our family frequently rode with him in his chauffeured limousine to visit Chinese farmers on their lush *fincas* (farms).

While he chatted with them, we happily feasted on *arroz con pollo* (saffron rice and chicken), avocado-pineapple salad and mango ice cream. I also remember Chinese shop-keepers inviting us to multi-course Chinese banquets. Between delicious courses, Father played the drinking game of scissors-paper-stone with his hosts. Losers had to drink up; soon rum led them to make so many mistakes they collapsed in a laughing heap. No wonder he was popular with his constituents. Although he worked hard, Father thoroughly enjoyed his job. He often said that China was so weak his requests did not carry the same weight as those of ambassadors from strong countries such as America. On the other hand, far from his homeland he could enjoy considerable independence to act as he thought best.

On Sundays we liked to drive along the broad seaside Malecon road that led past a picturesque lighthouse on a cliff. However, I had heard terrible stories about the lighthouse, so every time I saw it looming ahead, I shuddered as I visualized how Spanish soldiers used to push hapless Cuban prisoners into the shark-strewn waters below.

Some evenings we went to the popular San Souci café where people of all walks of life gathered. Beer flowed freely from a tap in the wall, while brown-skinned couples danced the rumba played by an enthusiastic, perspiring Cuban band. My parents neither danced nor drank beer. Instead they moved about the crowds to get to know the public, and socialize with friends and officials. They also wanted us youngsters to have informal contacts outside the legation, so we tagged along the whole evening. Feeling important, we would not have missed this opportunity for anything! Even today whenever I hear the strains of *La Cucaracha* (The Cockroach Song) I can still imagine the lively scenes at San Souci.

But best of all, I delighted in the splendid evening legation parties. Before each party, my parents spent days choosing a guest list of two to three hundred people. Then Mother called a few women friends and their cooks to help. For at least three days, they carefully prepared cold dishes to put on an enormous long dining room table, covered with a snow-white damask tablecloth and decorated with gleaming silver cutlery, candlesticks and bowls of flowers. On the night of the party, my brother, sister and I were fed early. Mother admonished, "Behave yourselves! Stay up here. You may peek through the banisters to watch the festivities below, but keep very quiet." With my head wedged between the stair posts at the top of the curving stairway, I had a great view of glittering glass chandeliers, gold painted furniture and brocade covered chairs vividly reflected in the large wall mirrors of the floor below. The glowing candles on the dining room table displayed an array of tempting, colorful dishes.

I was thrilled to watch the arriving guests—handsome black-mustached men in white tuxedos with gorgeously gowned and bejeweled ladies on their arms. I remember Father saying some of these men had violent pasts, since bloody feuds and revolts had been a fact of life in troubled Cuba for many years. The government could not control the turmoil and was even affected itself by corruption and abuses. He said with a sigh, "I hope in time these men will find peaceful ways to settle their differences."

But none of these misgivings showed at the party. My father regaled the guests with humorous stories as he filled their champagne glasses, or ordered more Bacardi rum to replenish their empty daiquiri glasses. Mother, resplendent in an embroidered mandarin gown, floated regally among the guests, greeting each by name, asking about their children, and inviting them to taste the dishes on the table. Mother's poise was astonishing. I felt so proud of them both. The sounds of excited Spanish chatter rose as the evening wore on. The laughter and clinking glasses wafted up the stairs, as we sleepy children eventually trailed off to bed.

At the end of our fourth year in Cuba, Father worriedly told us that a military coup was taking place against the government. Muffled bombs and gunshots sounded in the distance all day and into the night. Mother insisted, "No school for now." One night, shortly after midnight, the front gate doorbell rang. We heard whispers, followed by footsteps going upstairs to the third floor bedroom. The next morning, I was surprised to find our new occupant was none other than "Uncle" Carlos Saladrigas, Secretary of State. We all liked this tall, kindly, bespectacled gentleman, a special friend of Father's, who frequently came to dinner and talked politics into the night.

Father cautioned severely, "Tell no one that Uncle Saladrigas is here! He has political asylum, which means he is safe from people chasing him as long as he remains in this legation. But it's best if no one knows he is here." We readily promised. I didn't understand what was transpiring, but excitedly watched the daily food trays that went up, and our father's trips upstairs that sometimes lasted hours. After almost two months, Father told us the coup had failed and the government had regained its power. The shooting stopped and we were allowed to return to school. Shortly afterward, "Uncle" Saladrigas smilingly waved good-bye as he left the legation. As I waved back, I wondered how he would fare. For a time at least, the Cuban government recovered its stability.

A year later, Father finished his tour of duty and we returned to China. The incredible five years in Cuba still have a dream-like, unreal quality. Never again did I feel like a princess in a palace. But I was no longer wary of strange lands and peoples. Little did I realize how useful this attitude would soon be.

Chapter 4

NANJING AND SHANGHAI:
HOPE AND DESPAIR 1935-41

After five years in Cuba, we returned to live in Nanjing[5]. Father rented a comfortable, two-story house on top of a hill with a pleasant view of surrounding small farms. My younger sister and I entered the local grade school. Although I sensed I would need to reacquaint myself with Chinese ways, I was not prepared for the jolting switch from the elite multinational English-speaking private school we just left to this middle class Chinese-speaking school.

My Chinese was so rusty, a few students made fun of me saying, "You are a *wye guo-ren* (foreigner)." Aghast, I determined to change this. I switched from dresses to blue cotton Chinese long-gowns, became adept with chopsticks when eating the school lunches of rice, fish and vegetables, and studied hard to improve my Chinese. The turning point came when several classmates taught me colloquial terms, local ways and customs, and started to defend me against criticism. Gradually I was fully accepted—sharing secrets during recess.

---

[5] Nanjing: Capital of Republic of China, 150 miles inland from the coast in central China.

I recall several surprises during the transition. One was seeing a classmate with tiny needles stuck around her face to decrease headaches and menstrual cramps. Father said he preferred the Western medical view that acupuncture treatments did not have scientific basis. But my classmates countered that although they didn't know how, they claimed it did work, and they had no qualms in using it. Confronted with these conflicting opinions, I decided not to criticize, but to watch for treatment results. The results were variable.

I also remember vigorously championing Christianity to my Buddhist classmates. At twelve, I really didn't understand the basis of Christianity, so could not explain why there were so many competing divisions all trying to covert the Chinese. Nor could I explain why non-Christians could not enter heaven—assigning most of the Chinese to this fate. Actually, I didn't believe a fair God would do such a thing. Instead, I counter-attacked by asking why Buddhists didn't believe in God, since everyone knew that some great power created us. This silenced them for a while.

On the other hand, we were unified in our admiration for a fiery, young revolutionary history teacher. She shouted, "It is shameful that China lost the Opium Wars of 1840s against foreign powers. That loss contributed to China's decline." Fixing her eye on each of us, she demanded, "Today, China needs a vigorous central government to make her strong. Then she can once again take her rightful place in the world. Will each of you work hard for this?" Swayed by this pretty, dramatic young woman, we all shouted, "Yes!" These activities helped me reconnect to my Chinese cultural and political ties and finally feel a part of China again.

I enjoyed quiet, simple Nanjing. In spring, the nearby hills were fragrant with cherry blossoms. In summer, piles of mouth-watering watermelons were trucked in from Father's small farm. Oh, how I enjoyed lounging in the tiny teahouses aboard barges that leisurely floated between pink water lilies. When in season, friends gathered at our house to share steaming, boiled fresh crabs, which we dipped in small dishes of vinegar, soy sauce and chopped ginger, an unforgettable succulent taste! Mother often gave small dinner parties for Father's friends and government officials and allowed us youngsters to join. At the table I raptly listened to grown-ups discuss politics, economics and social concerns that stimulated and broadened my understanding of events of the time.

Most of our guests felt the nation was improving. Our leader, General Chiang, was keeping things relatively stable. Father worked in the Foreign Ministry building, an efficient-looking complex of unpretentious brick. Representing the country, he went on missions to Thailand (previously Siam) and Russia (previously the Soviet Union). He returned with fascinating tales, and wonderful gold and ivory gifts from the King of Siam. Not only was China slowly working its way up, but our family also seemed in comfortable circumstances. In a burst of confidence, Father began building our first home on the outskirts of the city. I remember the outside of a large building going up, and the still unfinished interior. Every day he visited the site. He boasted he was lining the closets with expensive and prized camphor wood, and putting in shower stalls and the most modern heating units.

It would have been a beautiful home, but we were never to live in it.

Our tranquility was shattered on a summer day in 1937. Father came home early, quietly conferred with Mother in his study, then emerged grim-faced to announce, "Japan has invaded China from the north. Her armies are marching toward us even now. Since our weak air force can't defend our skies, we are sure to be bombed. All families of government officials are ordered to leave the city within twenty-four hours. All other civilians must leave as soon as possible." His ominous words turned me cold. "What shall we do?" we asked. Father wanted us to go to Hongkong, an English controlled island far at the southern tip of China, but Mother thought that was too far. She preferred to take us children to stay with her sister's family in Shanghai, about one-hundred-fifty miles east. She thought if the military skirmish was over by late summer, she could bring us back in time for school. Father doubted the latter, but liked having us nearby. He also knew Mother would feel more comfortable among her relatives. He added, "Don't worry about me. I will stay with the government and I'll be careful."

The next morning, Mother and we three youngsters, each carrying a small suitcase of belongings, boarded a train to go live with our relatives in Shanghai. Although bewildered by the sudden change, I reassured myself that we would be back soon. This was not to be.

At first, we only saw life on the campus of St. John's University[6] where my uncle was vice-president. His family consisted of my aunt, a sweet-faced, hospitable woman, five daughters of about our ages, and innumerable cats. The house was always full of an assortment of relatives and university students—we never sat down to a supper table of less than twelve. They lived in a large, rambling house on the campus grounds. We were familiar with campus living, and got on well with our five cousins. Sleeping on makeshift cots in crowded bedrooms didn't bother us teenagers; in fact, we thought it was a lark.

---

[6]   St. John's University: an excellent Episcopal mission school in Shanghai. It included high school, and college undergraduate and graduate schools.

To my joy, I discovered an American missionary woman living on campus who owned bookshelves of children's stories in English. Hungry for adventure stories, I gobbled them up, shelf by shelf. The only title I still remember is the *Bobsey Twins* series; these books carried me into a world of happy children. In the process, I learned much useful English.

Perhaps I escaped into fantasy to mitigate the frightening war news of Chinese forces in full retreat, unable to fight the much stronger Japanese army. By midsummer, the entire Nationalist Government, and Father with them, moved to Chongqing, a Sichuan province city a thousand miles west. Nanjing fell to the Japanese, who committed terrible atrocities, including burning our house down and slaughtering our caretaker. All of our family assets, such as the house, deeds and bank accounts disappeared. Then followed ten cruel war years of inflation, poverty and suffering for the people.

That autumn, my brother returned to St. John's High School, and my sister and I entered St. Mary's High School, a sister school, because Mother believed we were safer in mission schools.

To ease the burden on my aunt's family, we moved into a small apartment in the French Concession, a special area in Shanghai controlled by the French. Our stay in Shanghai continued under a mounting pall of fear. Mother gave us dire warnings:

- Never tell anyone your father's occupation, since relatives of government officials are in much danger.
- Whenever you see a Japanese soldier on the streets, run and hide immediately, for they can take you away forever.
- Avoid crowds; they can be dangerous.
- Come directly home from school; don't loiter.
- Always dress simply, so you won't attract thieves, pickpockets or kidnappers.

We obeyed her implicitly, knowing our lives could depend on it. On the way to school, we passed pathetic refugees begging for food. Dead babies were often left on the streets, wrapped in newspapers. It was heartbreaking. When rice shipments came in, I saw riots in front of the rice shop. Overhead, Japanese war planes threatened, unchallenged.

Mother tried desperately to keep our family safe and functioning, and to this day I don't know how she did it. The Japanese army controlled areas between Shanghai and Chongqing, so she could get no word to or from Father and had to make all decisions alone. She hoarded scarce soap, salt, jam and canned milk. She kept a large cooking pot on the stove, into which she placed a big beef bone in water, adding any bits of meat, vegetables or rice she could find. This nourishing soup satisfied our daily hunger pangs. Thank goodness none of us became sick.

I recall feeling a great deal of free-floating fear, mainly of some outside threat of violence. But Mother's reassuring presence, my youth's optimism of "it can't happen to me," and my ignorance of the full situation shielded me from excessive worry. Threatening as it was, we went daily by foot and bus to school. I enjoyed my school friends and even exchanged visits with them. For a short time, a small elderly Chinese tutor came twice a week to teach us Chinese classics. This regular routine helped create the illusion of normalcy. Although I knew we had abruptly become poor, Mother's resourcefulness kept us from suffering.

But then the situation worsened. The Japanese easily occupied Shanghai. Luckily they wanted to preserve its important shipping activities, so it was more an administrative takeover than a military conquest. Nevertheless, Japanese soldiers took over police functions—a frightening act. The French Concession area was initially left unchanged, but we knew it would only be a matter of time before it too would be absorbed. Mother moved us again, this time to a small house surrounded by a high wall and guarded by a strong gate. She often kept us at home from school when she felt the streets were unusually dangerous. Some nights, angry people pounded on our gate, shouting to let them in. Mother told us to ignore the noise and go to sleep, and reassured us that the gate would hold.

We knew she was very worried when we heard her muttering, "I must get the girls out." She tried unsuccessfully to contact my father by sneaking messages through the surrounding enemy lines. She conferred with a few close friends and returned with a sober face. I awoke several nights in the dark to find her leaning over me, holding a lamp in one hand, and smoothing my hair with the other, as she anxiously gazed down at me.

After weeks of worried behavior, she suddenly became more cheerful. Gathering us around, she announced that my sister and I had received a scholarship to study at a small college in America, and she was sending us there. We gaped in astonishment. Over the next days she told us many good things about America, how we would be safe there and how we would have opportunities to study. She added that she and my brother would follow soon.

With this single decision, she changed my life forever.

Chapter 5

EASTWARD HO:
SAILING TO AMERICA 1941

On a cool, foggy spring morning in 1941, the ship's booming horn signaled departure from the Shanghai pier. I stared down from the ship's deck at the few people waving good-bye on the deserted pier. Normally, the pier was crowded with people, but this was war time; no one was traveling. Mother, standing alone, small and straight, black hair pulled into a bun at the back of her head, in her dark blue mandarin gown, was waving a white handkerchief. I was startled to see her usually smiling face streaming with tears!

My joy and excitement at leaving for America evaporated. In sudden dismay I stopped laughing and dancing as I gripped the ship's railing. At seventeen, I felt grown up going away with my younger sister to a new land. But at that moment, I realized I would be leaving Mother, the central figure in my life! Who would I run to with troubles? Who would guide me? Worse yet, would I ever see her again? What if she was killed? What if I failed in America? We had never talked about these problems. Mother just said, "Do your best. You will be safe in America. Things will turn out well." I burst into tears; my sister, not quite understanding, followed suit.

As the ship began to move, I shouted, "Wave to Ma-ma!" We both waved vigorously at the diminutive figure on the pier, which became smaller and smaller, and then disappeared. The huge American *SS President Cleveland* slowly and quietly slipped from war-torn China to head across the Pacific Ocean.

Having crossed the ocean before with our parents, we were familiar with bunk beds, portholes, dining room tables, deck walks and a daily schedule of activities. Our Asian features, straight bobbed black hair, full-length cotton mandarin gowns and passable English brought curious looks from other passengers, primarily returning Americans. In answer to many questions I replied, "Our mother is sending us to Virginia to study at Blackstone College for Girls. She wants us to escape danger from Japanese soldiers. She also said that in these troubled times, the best thing she can give us is a good education, so we can stand on our own feet." I added, "We learned English from our mother and in St. Mary's mission school in Shanghai. Mother's missionary friend will meet us in San Francisco, to put us on a train to Virginia." Then standing straight, I proudly announced, "I am the older one, so I am responsible for both of us."

The next morning the loudspeaker blared, "Ladies and gentlemen, please ready yourselves to stop overnight at this Japanese port for the ship to fuel and take aboard supplies. Those disembarking will go through passport control." This unexpected stop-over threw me into a panic. Japan was the home of our enemy! Mother had warned us to avoid any contact with the Japanese. Might soldiers come aboard and whisk us away?

When I asked other passengers, they laughed, "No, no, they will not do that." But could I trust these strangers? In a quandary, I finally decided we should lock ourselves in our cabin and ignore any knocks on the door. I pocketed some bread rolls, asked for a thermos of tea and double locked the door.

My sister remonstrated, "How would the Japanese know we are on board? We can't hurt them. Why would they want to take us away?"

"I'm not taking any chances," I told her. "We must not go outside our cabin." For a while, I even convinced her to hide under the beds. But this became too stuffy and uncomfortable, so we crawled out to tensely sit all afternoon. That evening we finished our meager stash of bread and tea, and lay down for the night. We did not unlock the door until the ship was safely on its way.

Mother's missionary friend, "Aunt" Minta, met us in San Francisco, put us and our two trunks on a train and carefully instructed the conductor to watch over us during the cross-country trip. The train chugged over high mountains, broad plains, miles of farmlands and into several large cities, where it briefly stopped. Knowing little American geography, I could not identify the scenes that rushed by, but the enormous size of the country took my breath away. Days and nights passed in a haze. As my excitement died down, I began to think about this pivotal turning point in my life, and reviewed the things Mother told us, trying to understand its full implications.

I was truly independent now. For the first time in my life, I was completely on my own. I would have to make my own decisions big and small, from handling our scanty finances to when to cut my hair. Mother, across the ocean, could no longer help me. If my younger sister asked for advice, I would have to try to offer it. Never having done any of this before, I was not sure I could. But since Mother must have had confidence in me, I resolved to do my best.

"America," Mother had said, "is a country of friendly people and clean streets. Ordinary people have a far better standard of living than we can imagine. Laws govern all activities, and people are mostly law-abiding. The people follow Christian ethical standards; most are regular church-goers. Young people go to school because they know that the better educated they are, the better jobs they can get and the more money they will earn to have a good life. I want you to succeed in these new ways." She added, "Best of all, you don't have to be afraid anymore. In America, the laws, society and Christian standards will protect you. People are judged by who they are and what they do, not by their father's place in society, so if you work hard and follow the rules you will succeed."

I mulled over these ideas; they were so different from all that I had experienced in China. Ever since the war with Japan, I had been afraid—of violence, of hunger, of being lost, of chaos. I had been afraid to speak freely, or to act in any way that would attract the attention of authorities. I knew that once jailed I would have no recourse to get free again. To my parents I meant a great deal, but to society I meant nothing. Could I really be free of these fears in America? It was almost too much to believe. Mother's assertion that I would be judged by what I said and did, rather than who my father was seemed impossible. Could I really count as a person on my own?

I accepted any success would come through education and training, just as it had for my parents. Contrary to most Chinese at that time who did not believe in educating daughters, my parents brought us up believing girls and boys had equal potential and should be equally prepared with a good, sound education. But Mother had sadly added, "I have no money to help you, so you will have to get scholarships to go to school. That means you will have to excel with good grades." Although I had not yet decided on a goal, I was determined to study hard.

Having decided these weighty matters, I relaxed and concentrated on learning what I could from my trip. I gazed at the passing scenery, listened to fellow passenger's conversations, enjoyed the meals in the dining car, slept soundly in the bunks and engaged in the usual give-and-take with my sister. "It's ten o'clock and time for bed," I would say. "No, not yet, it's too early," she would say. "You know Mother always had us in bed by ten. We must do what she thought best." Reluctantly my sister would agree. Time passed quickly.

One morning the black porter making up our bunks asked where we were going. When I replied we were going to a Virginia college to study, he looked at me strangely and said, "You folks come from China to study at a white college here, but even though I'm born here I can't." I would ponder these words in the ensuing years while I lived in the South.

We arrived at the small town of Blackstone, Virginia on a warm sunny afternoon. The air was filled with the fragrance of dogwood, the tree branches heavy with delicate white and pink blossoms. It was lush and green everywhere. Anxiously we waited at the quiet little train station until an elderly black man in overalls, sitting on a cart drawn by a horse, stopped to ask, "Going to Blackstone College, Miss?" At our "yes," he piled our luggage onto his cart, and we started toward the college. The leisurely pace of the horse and the easy manner of the man calmed our tense nerves.

About twenty minutes later, we turned a corner to see a stately colonial-style college building. Nearly every one of the two hundred girls of the school seemed to be hanging out the windows waiting for a glimpse of us. Many said we were the first Asians they had ever seen. Soon my sister and I were ensconced on two beds in our assigned dormitory room, surrounded by jabbering girls. Peppered with eager questions, we answered as best we could.

"Yes, we had a pleasant trip." "Yes, we like what we see of America." "No, we were not molested by Japanese soldiers." "We wear Chinese gowns because that is all we have." "Our trunks only contain more gowns." "No, we don't know anything about the latest dance in America." "Yes, we would like to see it." The room was promptly cleared and four girls demonstrated jitterbugging and the *Big Apple* to our amused delight.

That was how my sister and I entered this Promised Land—with a trunk of clothes and fifty dollars each.

Chapter 6

GETTING TO KNOW AMERICA:
VIRGINIA & MASSACHUSETTS 1941-45

My Americanization could not have begun more smoothly or in a gentler environment than at Blackstone College for Girls. Farmers and shop-keepers sent their daughters to this small Methodist high school and junior college to be educated and learn to be ladies. Located in a typical sleepy Southern town, it escaped the crowding and tensions of large cities. The warm climate and flowering trees created a sheltered spot for young women to grow to maturity.

The girls in their late teens were cheerful, carefree and fun-loving. Treating us as exotic foreigners, they introduced us to many American ways amid giggles and laughter. "Silly, don't bow, just speak up to people." "Try pinning up your hair with bobby pins." My fears of external violence receded as I embraced this new country and its people.

The spacious college building had classrooms and administrative offices on the ground floor and dormitory rooms on the upper two floors. My sister and I shared a large room with two friendly girls. The principal decided the first priority was for us to obtain high school diplomas, so he started my sister as a junior and me as a senior in high school. During the week, we attended three to four classes a day, and on weekends we played field hockey and attended Sunday service at a nearby Methodist church.

My teachers in English Literature and History of Western Civilization created excitement for me. I can still see the two friends who were often together—slim, young women dressed in stylish, subdued-colored dresses, irresistibly passionate about their subjects. The English teacher introduced me to the beauty of the language, and the works of literary giants such as Shakespeare, Wordsworth, Poe and Dickinson. Even today when I hear their words quoted, I feel a familiar thrill of pleasure. To study for her class, I read English classics in the school library; although half understood, I still enjoyed their sheer beauty. The history teacher led me through the development of the English-speaking people in Western Europe, from the time of the ancient Greeks to the nineteenth century. The endless violent wars of kings reminded me of Chinese history. Out of this European cauldron came America.

In American Civics class, I saw how various wars, together with political and legal decisions, created this country. For the first time I began to understand what a true democracy was. This was an astonishing new concept for me, coming from a country that had never held elections. I was deeply moved to learn that in America the government represented the people, and it was the people who made the changes when it was in their best interest—truly a nation ". . . of the people, by the people and for the people . . . ."[7] I could scarcely believe my good fortune to live where these principles were put into practice.

Although the classes were easy, I found them so engrossing that I studied hard and graduated from high school with good

---

[7]   President Lincoln's Gettysburg address, November 19, 1863

grades. In junior college, my sister and I also did well; we even began tutoring fellow students. With delighted amazement we realized we had good minds; we could seriously consider higher education and a profession. I graduated junior college magna cum laude; my sister did equally well a year later.

As a scholarship student, I worked at various school jobs. Half the students were on scholarships, so we worked together to keep the school functioning. I discovered that work had dignity here; unlike in China, I could work at anything honest, including manual work, without dishonoring myself. What a relief and challenge, I thought. I was assigned to assist the dietitian, a tiny, weather-beaten woman of uncertain age, who managed the kitchen and dining room with an iron hand. She started me waiting on student tables, later at the principal's table and finally in a most important position as her assistant. My first lesson concerned diets, that we must eat a daily balance of proteins, carbohydrates, fruits and vegetables. Once convinced of its truth, I have since followed it diligently for myself and others. In that large kitchen, I soon became familiar with carcasses of meat, five-pound cans of vegetables, sacks of potatoes and as much fresh fruits as could fill the shelves and refrigerators. After seeing near famine conditions in China, this abundance stunned me. Daily I watched the diminutive dietitian and the huge cook scurrying around the kitchen to produce healthy, tasty meals for the entire school. I was proud to help in this significant effort.

In addition, my sister and I found ways to earn pocket money for modest expenses. We started a newspaper route in the dormitory, getting up an hour before class to deliver papers to subscriber's doorsteps. Near winter holidays we sold Christmas cards. When other girls went home for short holidays, we stocked merchandise on shelves of the local Five-and-Ten store. We were elated to earn our own money for the first time in our lives.

On a December afternoon, we huddled around a radio to hear President Roosevelt declare, "Yesterday, December 7, 1941– a date which will live in infamy–the United States of America was suddenly and deliberately attacked by naval and air forces of the Empire of Japan."[8] This Pearl Harbor attack began America's war with Japan and Germany. I had a sinking feeling at the thought of another war. We were anxious for the safety of my mother and brother in Shanghai. What a relief when we received Mother's letter that described their trip on one of the last passenger ships crossing the Pacific. We felt Father was safe in Chongqing, the Chinese government's wartime stronghold.

She wrote that my brother had enrolled at Washington University Medical School, St. Louis, and when he volunteered for the armed forces he was placed in the Reserve Officer Training Corp (ROTC). She said, "Since all of you are in school, and I can't afford to stay near you doing nothing, I may as well stay with my friends in California. Perhaps I can get a job to pay my way." Shortly afterward, she started in a factory sewing silk parachutes for the U.S. Air Force and developed an interest in work place labor laws. How like Mother, I thought with a smile, to come up a winner.

Surprisingly, World War II had relatively little impact on our school life. Because of rationing, my sister and I looked forward to weekend invitations to my roommate's farm, where we could gorge on meat, butter and ice cream. Our college held a few carefully supervised dances for the "boys in uniform" stationed at a nearby army camp. As we awkwardly stumbled around on the dance floor, I told them how afraid I was for them on the battlefield, and they told me how they envied my

---

8   War message to Congress, December 8, 1941.

freedom to study. I was profoundly grateful that in spite of the war, my sister and I continued to live and study in an untroubled environment, so different from previous life in Shanghai.

Two other women stood out in my memory of those times—the first was Mrs. Dunn. Shortly after arrival at the school, we were told a lady from town was downstairs asking to see us. A plump, brown-haired, middle-aged woman greeted us with the friendliest, widest smile I had ever seen. Her sparkling brown eyes, patrician features and whole being seemed concentrated in that smile.

"Honey," she said with a lilting Southern accent, "I'm Mrs. Dunn. My husband is one of the two doctors here. Years ago, I spent six unforgettable months as a missionary in China. Now I want to welcome you both to Blackstone." She asked about our trip and how we were settling in, then invited us to visit her home. We were apparently taken under her wing.

I recall many a cool afternoon sitting by her crackling fire roasting marshmallows. She attentively listen without comment while we poured out feelings and observations. We needed adult reassurance and she was there for us. I was fascinated by her easy elegance and her unconventional speech and ways. For example, she said with a laugh, "My left face is more attractive, so I always turn that side to my husband." She treated black people as equals when this was not done in the South. She won my love and admiration for her kindness, generosity and unmatched zest for life. Because she had taught French, we called her "La Dunn."

During our first summer in Blackstone, she took us to a YWCA Girl's Camp for eight-to-twelve-year-old girls, and dubbed me the "drama counselor." In the mornings I combed and braided the girls' hair, in the afternoons I taught them little skits and at night I guided them with a flashlight to the outhouse when they wakened me with, "I gotta go." Whenever the evening sky was clear, we sat in a circle around a campfire, and La Dunn led us in storytelling and song. Sometimes, as a treat, we were allowed to wrap ourselves in blankets and fall asleep under the stars. What a lovely introduction to America for a foreign city girl!

La Dunn urged me to always look my best. "Honey, hold your head high and look people in the eye. Stand up straight and stick your tail feathers out." When she saw me smile she said, "You have an attractive smile. Do smile often." She liked my simple wardrobe, "Wear blue, you look good in it," and approved of my good grades, "Fine, you have a brain. Use it to serve others." She always had nice things to say about how I looked and dressed—something nobody had ever done before. I had felt plain and unattractive until she made me feel otherwise. Shyness and tenseness left me in her presence. This new confidence, so important to a young woman, has stayed with me ever since. Although we were separated after I left Blackstone, we kept in touch by phone and letters. La Dunn remained my dear friend, confidant and guiding spirit for the rest of her life.

The other woman, whose name I no longer recall, was my mathematics teacher who opened another side of American life to us. An awkward, earnest young woman from Boston, she had come to teach at Blackstone and then met and married a handsome local farmer. She invited my sister and me to spend our summer vacation on her farm. In return for room and board, we would help with physical chores. For two months we worked the long hours required to run a farm. At daybreak we women fed and watered the chickens, then cultivated the vegetable garden. During the afternoons we washed, cleaned and spent hours standing over a hot stove "canning" or bottling vegetables and fruits for the winter. How our fingers stiffened, our arms hurt, our backs ached and our feet swelled toward evening. Her husband rode the tractor all day, yet could wise-crack and tease at supper. To me, he epitomized the sturdy, resilient American farmer. After supper, we would briefly read books or newspapers, then fall exhausted into bed. I never again took food lightly, remembering what hard work it was to produce it.

In Blackstone, I encountered my first experience with the Southern racial problem. Meeting groups of black people was new to me. They comprised about a third of the town population and kept it going by performing many essential jobs, but were so quiet they seemed invisible. My surprise came one day while boarding a local bus. As I sat down in front, the bus driver curtly ordered me, "Go sit in the back of the bus."

"But I'm not black, I'm Chinese."

After taking a careful look at my straight hair and Chinese clothes, he said, "Okay, you can sit up front."

My schoolmates had warned me to use only bathrooms and drinking fountains labeled "White" and avoid those labeled "Black." When I finally realized that black people were considered second class citizens, I was puzzled and tried to discuss the issue, but to my surprise, no one wanted to. I regret now that I did not push for explanations.

Two other circumstances involving black people left a favorable impression. On warm evenings at school, after supper clean-up chores, the black cooks, maids and cleaning people sat in a circle on the ground outside and spontaneously sang songs in perfect multi-part harmony—a wonderful sound I had never heard before. I marveled at this extraordinary natural musical talent. Another place where my sister and I met them was in their churches. Both black and white churches invited us to talk about China, and their congregations were equally kind and courteous. We welcomed the chance to get acquainted with people in the community; moreover, we loved the

Southern-style fried chicken dinners. In contrast to the five or ten dollars in an envelope that white congregations handed us, the black congregation usually took an offering, showering the collection plate with dollar bills that often added up to near thirty dollars. I was touched by such generosity from people who had so little!

After two and a half years at Blackstone, I was sufficiently confident to plan a career. Because of the war, I abandoned the idea of becoming a teacher like my mother, and decided a nurse would be more useful when I returned to China. When I discussed this with my brother, who was already in medical school, I remember his answer well.

"Oh no," he said, "Go for medicine. You can do so much more as a doctor."

"But brother," I replied, "I don't have the brains to be a doctor."

"Nonsense, medicine is ten percent brains, ninety percent perspiration. You can do it." Hard work had never been a problem for me. Without further ado, I decided to become a doctor. A lifetime decision, made in a flash, surprisingly turned out to be just right.

I realized that a school record from an obscure college would not help me in the keen competition to get into a good medical school. Moreover, I still needed many premedical science courses not available at Blackstone. I applied for a two-year scholarship to cover these sciences at Mt. Holyoke College in Massachusetts—one of the "big four" prestigious east coast women colleges. My good grades must have helped, because to my delight I was accepted. A year later, my sister was accepted by Bryn Mawr College, Pennsylvania to take biochemistry. From then our paths diverged as we followed different career paths. Although I missed our companionship, I was happy each of us felt free to create our own lives.

The six-year climb to become a doctor began in earnest. The basic sciences included biology, physics, biochemistry and trigonometry. The physics teacher expected us to find solutions to his "magic" demonstrations in class. Biochemistry introduced us to electrons and protons. I barely passed trigonometry.

Biology intrigued me as I learned about the organs in the body and their functions, but the corresponding laboratory class both fascinated and repelled me. While following the development of a fertilized chicken egg, I marveled to discover that the chick embryo in the yolk looked much like a human embryo—evidence that we started as simple forms, then differentiated into more complex higher forms. On the other hand, biology dissection repelled me. Perched on a high stool over a laboratory table, I looked down on a recently dead frog, lying on his back in a metal pan, awaiting my dissecting knife. The frog's skin was cold and clammy to touch; it smelled of dank mildew; its bulging eyes stared accusingly at me. What was I to do? I gritted my teeth, swallowed, lowered my scalpel and began to mechanically follow the teacher's instructions.

But these required subjects paled beside the fascinating non-science classes. Excellent teachers in this fine college laid before me a whole new world. I attended or audited these classes with the thirst of a wanderer who found water in the desert—ancient history, political science, philosophy, etc., as many as the dean would allow.

My blind political science teacher came to class with a seeing-eye dog to guide a lively debate on Great Britain giving independence to India. A brilliant, lumbering history teacher from Eastern Europe brought Greek and Roman history alive. He showed us the Athenians gathered to hear classic Greek plays in the hillside theatre in the shadow of the Parthenon temple; we saw Socrates drink the cup of hemlock poison when accused of defiling youths with his philosophical teachings. We thrilled to Roman legions marching in phalanx as they conquered the known western world, and we feasted with Romans reclining on couches tasting foods from all corners of the empire. Our class voted the Roman era the period in the past we would most like to have lived in.

Unexpectedly, I found it stimulating to get to know and talk to many thoughtful schoolmates. These girls were different from those at Blackstone; they were daughters of professional and business people who expected them to perform well and amount to something in society, whether as mothers or as professionals. I could not get enough of the late night jamborees, as we sat around in pajamas on dormitory beds talking about everything, including philosophy, men, family, politics, the war and so on, long into the night. The future seemed full of exciting possibilities.

As a scholarship student, I helped run our cooperative house. I recall, with amusement, that one of the jobs was to ring the wake-up bell at seven o'clock. I was so afraid of oversleeping and the girls missing their classes, that I set three separate alarm clocks around my bedroom, and dashed around turning them off each morning. Outside the house, my jobs were to clean glassware in various laboratories and help set up experiments. Although these jobs were light work, they ate up time. In the time left I diligently studied to keep up my vital grades. At the end of two years, I graduated with a BA degree, and was pleased to be invited to join the Phi Beta Kappa Honorary Scholastic Society.

My college years not only introduced me to this wonderful country, but in these years I mastered my basic science courses, and in addition had exposure to liberal arts courses that broadened and deepened my whole life. Now more focused challenges awaited.

Chapter 7

MICHIGAN:
TOUGH MEDICAL SCHOOL
YEARS 1945-49

I n the fall of 1945, I began four years of medical school at
the University of Michigan. My world suddenly
narrowed. From eight in the morning until five in the afternoon
a torrent of scientific and medical facts unceasingly poured into
my head.

Our first class started at seven-thirty in the morning in the
Anatomy Laboratory. About a hundred classmates and I
gathered outside Room A, and made nervous small talk. "Where
are you from?" "Which dorm do you live in?" "What do you
think we will do today?"

Suddenly a loud bell rang, and the door of Room A flew
open. We shoved into an enormous room, to see sunlight shining
through large, bare windows onto gray walls and a gray cement
floor. About twenty numbered tables were positioned at different
angles. On top of each table lay a long quiet shape covered with
a green-gray rubber sheet. Formaldehyde fumes burned my
eyes and nostrils. A kind-faced, white-haired professor wearing
a white lab coat called out our names and table numbers,
grouping us four to a table.

"Please uncover your tables," the professor directed.

Sudden gasps sounded throughout the room. Under each sheet, lay a blue-gray human cadaver, completely nude except for small towels laid over the head and pelvis.

"These are your cadavers," he declared, "to dissect the different areas we will cover in class. Two of you will work together on each side of the table. Please introduce yourselves to each other. You have one hour to dissect the major arteries in the forearms."

As I looked down at the cadaver, I felt an even stronger revulsion than I had with the frog in biology class—this was once a human being! After swallowing hard for a few minutes, I carried on. "Doing medicine" was going to be tough! I sincerely hoped I could make it.

In the first two years we covered anatomy, physiology, biochemistry, pathology, pharmacology, bacteriology and more. My main problem was fighting fatigue and sleep in order to master the enormous amount of data given. In the second year, I devised a study schedule for myself. At five o'clock after a day of lectures, I trudged to my dormitory for rest and supper. After supper, I reviewed the day's lectures then went to sleep from ten o'clock until my alarm woke me at four in the morning. Dragging myself from my warm bed, I squeezed in another two hours of study, then dropped off to sleep for an additional hour until the morning dormitory bell woke me at seven. The endless flow of facts, quizzes and exams were so demanding, I often wondered if I really belonged in this school.

I was the fortunate recipient of a Barbour Scholarship[9] to

---

9   Barbour Scholarship: scholarship program of Michigan University Graduate School, established by Levi L. Barbour in 1914 for the benefit of Oriental women.

which I owe my medical education. Its goal was to prepare Oriental women to serve their countries at home or abroad. It generously provided room, board and tuition, and required no work in compensation. To keep my scholarship and to show my appreciation for this opportunity, I made it a point to maintain a high grade point average. Since these medical students were the brightest people I had ever competed against, I was pushed to the limit of my mental ability. In the process, I learned what an extraordinary structure the human body is, and how remarkably well we function. My challenge as a doctor would be to help patients cope with hostile organisms, disease and aging.

Studying daily elbow-to-elbow with my classmates, I came to know them well, especially the dozen or so women in our class of about a hundred. At first, most of the men were on reserve status, so they marched smartly into class each morning wearing Army or Navy uniforms. After World War II ended during our second year, I was startled to see them in casual shirts and pants. Some glamour was lost, but it did allow me to become acquainted with the real persons. My classmates were a splendid bunch—dedicated, hard-working and kind—and I felt it a privilege to be among them. Phil, an outstanding student, was an accurate note-taker who started selling copies of his class notes to supplement his income. Two mornings after a class, we could buy a complete set of lecture notes to round-out and correct our fragmented personal copies. His notes were invaluable not only for their accuracy, but they freed us to concentrate more attentively on the lectures.

To my joy, the third and fourth years of medical school were clinical and much more relaxed. For the first time we started seeing patients in the hospital, heard practicing doctors give lectures in hospital seminar rooms and watched demonstrations at the patient's bedside. All the disparate scientific data of the past two years finally came together when I applied it to sick patients. The medical subjects fascinated me—medicine, surgery, pediatrics, neurology, psychiatry and later gynecology, obstetrics, eye, ear, nose and throat. I relished finally interacting with real people! Of course, every time we studied a new disease we were sure we had it, leading to many needless visits to the student health clinic. Our physician teachers thoroughly drilled us on the cause, probable mechanisms and symptoms of various disease entities, but only scantily covered treatment regimens. They explained, "You will learn the latest treatments as you follow your field. They will continually change and improve, but the basic understanding of disease states will always be the cornerstone of your work."

Syphilis and tuberculosis were the two scourges in medicine in those pre-antibiotic days. Because their symptoms at different disease stages could mimic almost any other disease, we had to study them thoroughly. Prevention was the key, since current treatments were ineffective—heavy metals injections for syphilis, and fresh air and bed rest for tuberculosis. My classmates and I routinely gowned, gloved and masked whenever we visited patients in the Tuberculosis Sanitarium at the edge of the university grounds, or when we handled tissues in the pathology laboratory. In spite of great care, however, in almost every class one or two students invariably came down with tuberculosis. In those days this meant life-long illness if not early death. The threat hung like a sword over our heads. With great luck my class was spared.

We learned the vital skill of taking a patient's history and doing a physical examination to form a diagnosis. My first test patient was a pleasant woman of fifty-four with an obscure, persistent backache. While a physician teacher observed my technique, I spent forty-five minutes taking her history and fifteen minutes completing a physical examination. I then summarized the pertinent facts to him, listing my "differential diagnoses" (list of possible diagnoses based on the findings) and requesting tests to exclude certain diagnoses and confirm the most likely one. Her history could not explain the pain, but my physical examination revealed an enlarged, hardened liver. Laboratory tests and X-rays revealed this to be a malignant lesion pressing on her spinal nerves causing her back pain. Although elated at arriving at the correct diagnosis, I was saddened to arrive at this death sentence. My aptness at diagnosis convinced me I could become a good internal medicine specialist.

During my first year in medical school I met my lifelong friend, Ruth, a law student. We were living in the same dormitory. Tall, strongly built, with a broad good-looking face and large penetrating brown eyes, Ruth moved quickly and decisively. Although always pleasant and polite, she had a no-nonsense air that brooked no frivolities or intrusion into her privacy. One night, after vainly seeking a quiet place to study a box of human bones (not possible in the library), I approached her. She answered, "Why, yes. I do odd jobs at the law quad, so I have keys to all the rooms. You could use one of the empty rooms if you like." I quickly accepted. This boon helped me pass the first difficult year.

Ruth put herself through law school by working at multiple jobs, including running the dormitory telephone switchboard. Her rigid schedule of work and study left little time for any contact except occasional talks over cups of tea. Gradually we learned to know each other and became firm friends. Our professional goals, meager incomes and wish to succeed in a man's world were common bonds. I especially admired her independence and drive, and realized she was a person I could depend on. Even after I left medical school, we visited each other periodically and encouraged each other's professional growth. She once said, "If I'm your friend, it will be for always." Years later, she proved this in unexpected ways.

The slackened pace of study in these last clinical years freed me to turn to long postponed extra-curricular activities. During the war years, the university had a large group of foreign graduate students not subject to the draft. Among the Chinese in this group, the men mostly majored in engineering or mathematics, and the women in chemistry. We socialized at monthly meetings of the Chinese student club, usually for potluck dinners and talk. To my surprise I was elected president one year. My only achievement was to organize a fashion show, where the women paraded in beautiful silk gowns to appreciative applause, especially from the men.

This led to a few dinner dates with other graduate students, mostly Chinese. At this my first coeducational school, I found men an interesting novelty. My most enduring friendships were with a Harvard medical student and a Michigan doctoral candidate in theoretical physics. Both were attractive Chinese men who honored me with marriage proposals. However, I was not really ready to think about marriage then, so I rationalized my indifference with superficial explanations to myself, that the budding physician was too spoiled and the physicist was too impractical. So I sadly said, "No" and we parted our ways.

A most important event was the Ling family reunion in New York City. Chosen to represent China in the International Monetary Conference at Bretton Woods, New Hampshire in 1944, Father was due to arrive in New York by plane. That July, Mother from California, my brother from Missouri, my sister from Pennsylvania and I from Massachusetts, joyfully converged at the New York International Airport. An American volunteer pilot in a small plane had carried Father "over the hump" (Himalayas and the Burma Road), across India, the Middle East and then to New York. Very thin, dressed in an old khaki shirt and pants, Father bounced down the airplane steps with a delighted grin. With tears and hugs we greeted each other after seven years of separation. Knowing many Chinese families were separated, or had members lost or killed, we were deeply grateful to be together again and in good health. Later, my parents settled in an apartment on the east side of Manhattan for easy access to conference sites. We three siblings then returned to our medical studies.

In 1949 the Chinese Communist Party defeated the Nationalist Government to take control of China. Father lost his government post and decided to retire and stay with Mother in New York. Following events in China, we were horrified to learn that Grandmother Ling had been killed by the Communists—beaten to death in a kangaroo court[10]—in its sweep to eliminate the landowner class. Father never forgave this cruelty; he would have no part of such a government. He said bitterly, "The Communists want you to 'Hate what you love, and love what you hate.'" He predicted they would cause the Chinese people untold suffering to maintain power.

Having my parents nearby again was a great relief. When I visited them during summer vacations, I could eat Mother's good cooking, enjoy discussions with them on my school progress and family affairs, and thrash out the events of the nation and the world. Father even tried to teach me something about stock investing. More than anything, however, I cherished their support and encouragement. "You are doing just fine. Continue as you are. Be sure to get enough rest. Can we send you any food?" And as always, I learned much from their wisdom.

---

[10] Kangaroo court: a mock court which illegally passes and executes judgement, said to be so named because its justice progresses by leaps and bounds.

I especially needed their guidance in the last hectic months before graduation, when I faced the dilemma of whether to return to China as previously planned or to stay in America for specialty training. My U.S. immigration status was in limbo—my student visa had expired and my application for permanent residency had stalled. Nearly all my fellow Chinese students were making arrangements to return.

"Come," they said, "the Communist government is settling down, and there is much work to do. You already know enough to practice good medicine in China."

But Father strenuously disagreed. He had no illusions about the Communists.

"No," he said emphatically, striking a fist into his open palm and pacing the floor, "Don't go now. Wait to see if they will change their ruthless ways. I understand your patriotic intentions, but you must be cautious."

"But Father, I will just quietly practice medicine, and not get involved in politics."

"Don't be naive," he said. "The Communists will not allow you to work in your own way. They will lock you in a re-education camp until you declare your support for their policies. You are so stubborn, I'm afraid they may never let you out."

Trusting his political judgment, I decided to delay my return until the picture became clearer. I proceeded to plan for specialty training in internal medicine. Looking back now, I realize Father had saved me from a fatal misstep. My colleagues who returned to China were suspect and not trusted because they had been in America. Not only were they not allowed to work in their field, but many were also deliberately humiliated by being forced to do menial labor. A bright young woman eye doctor who returned was later seen forced to carry luggage at a train station. Thank goodness I escaped this fate!

What a proud day it was for my parents and me, when resplendent in my blue-gold hood over black cap and gown, I was presented with the diploma of *Doctor of Medicine* in graduation ceremonies at the huge Michigan University football stadium. Completing one big step, I now faced another—internship and residency training. Delighted to enter this noble profession, I couldn't wait to practice what I had learned.

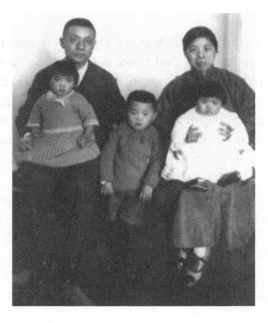

Ling family in Tianjin, China, 1925
(left to right) author at 2 yrs, with brother and sister

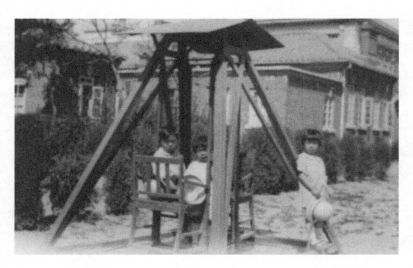

Author (standing) and siblings in Tianjin, China
Playground on Nankai University campus, 1928

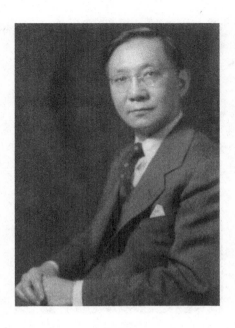

Author's father, Dr. Ping Ling, Chinese Minister to Cuba, 1932

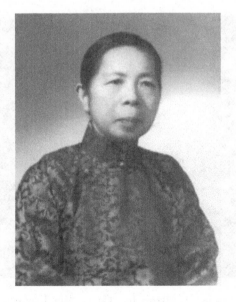

Author's mother, Mrs. Clara Ling, Havana, Cuba

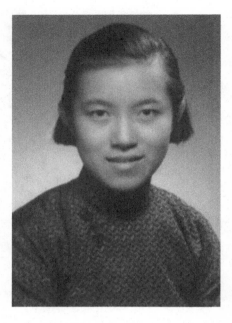

Author as school girl, Ling Kuo-fen, in Nanjing, China 1938

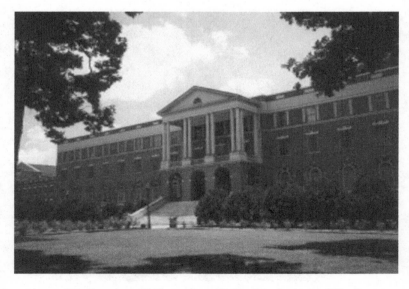

Blacktsone College for Girls, Blackstone, VA
(photo by Blackstone classmate Helen Garnett).

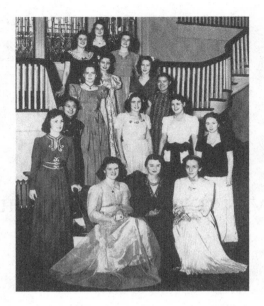

"Gable Girls" Students living in Blackstone College President's residence, the Gables, (author on right, sister on left of pyramid) From College Archives of Blackstone

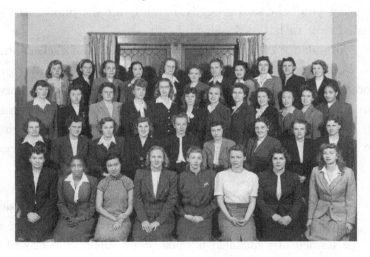

Women medical students, University of Michigan 1945-49 (author first row, third from left). Photo from Jane (Watson) Duncan-second row, fourth from left.

Chapter 8

MINNEAPOLIS:
EVEN TOUGHER INTERNSHIP
YEAR 1950

The phone rang at two a.m. in my tiny room over the Minneapolis General Hospital garage. Kate, my roommate, picked up the receiver next to her bed.

"For you," she said groggily, handing me the phone, as she turned over to fall back asleep.

"Ambulance call, Doc," a voice said, and then clicked off.

I quickly pulled on a white intern's[11] jacket and skirt over my underclothes, jumped into my shoes, grabbed my stethoscope and ran downstairs to the garage. The ambulance was already revving up as I donned the oversized intern's wool-lined parka hanging on a nail, picked up the heavy ambulance bag of medicines and

---

[11] Intern: a graduate M.D. physician in his/her first year of practice training after medical school. This one-year training period is performed in a qualified hospital under supervision of senior physicians, and is a requirement to obtain a medical license for general practice.

syringes, and leapt aboard. With lights flashing, our eerie siren shattered the silence as we sped through dark, empty streets.

Even after two months of this routine, I still couldn't suppress a chilling fear at each emergency call. Scenes of injuries and mangled bodies haunted me. What horror will it be this time? Will I quickly make the right critical decisions? At least the ambulance driver was an old pro, and a Minneapolis police squad car came along whenever possible. Their presence bolstered my confidence.

We stopped on a dark street in front of a two-story house with lights blazing. Flanked by the ambulance driver and a policeman, I entered the house lugging my medical bag. Two men and a woman led us to a couch. A fully dressed boy of about eleven was lying on his back, eyes closed. A gun lay on the floor by his side.

A wild-eyed woman rushed up, "This is Danny, my son. We heard a loud sound, like a shot, and I found him on the floor of his Dad's study. We moved him here with the gun, and called the ambulance. I can't wake him up," she ended with a wail.

The boy was not breathing. I could feel no carotid pulse at his neck. There was no sign of blood. I pulled up his shirt to listen for a heart beat, and saw a bullet hole just over his heart. Death must have been instantaneous.

I gently took the woman's hand, and told her that her son was gone. The room soon filled with the sounds of sobbing. Police questioning revealed Danny's father kept his gun locked in his office closet. Somehow the boy must have found it unlocked, started playing with the gun and accidentally shot himself. This was the police's preliminary conclusion, but he indicated further investigation would follow. As I rode back to the hospital in silence, I felt a heavy heart at another needless death.

On these runs we were sometimes lucky to find an injury or an infection we could treat on the spot or at the hospital. Even drunks that we pulled out of the gutter could be sobered up in the emergency room while we checked them for injuries. But bizarre and tragic conditions were not uncommon. These ambulance calls introduced me to a seamy, urgent and sometimes dangerous side of city life for which I was totally unprepared. I left a sheltered academic environment to enter this entirely different one. I was beginning to realize the heavy responsibility I now carried as a doctor. In crises and emergencies, decisions were always directed at me. "What should we do, Doc?" Ultimately, it was up to me.

A year of internship was required of all medical school graduates to earn a license to practice medicine. I chose to intern at this big city hospital, where I could get the widest variety of experiences. Every month or two I was "rotated" to a different service—medicine, surgery, pediatrics, obstetrics-gynecology, neurology, ear-nose-and-throat, or emergency room-ambulance service.

After graduating in June 1949 I arrived here on July first, with only theoretical and carefully supervised medical school training. I was issued a white uniform, assigned a room and a roommate, handed an intern call schedule and was expected to go forth to take care of Minneapolis' sickest and poorest. Ostensibly, we were supervised by the senior residents[12] of the

---

[12] Resident: a M.D. physician in a three-to-five year training program for a specialty after their internship. It is conducted in a qualified medical center under supervision of physician specialists. An Internal Medicine doctor specializes in problems of the heart, lungs, intestines, hormones, etc.

nearby University Hospital, who conducted morning rounds and advised us on the care of our patients. Actually they were often difficult to find, so in reality we were pretty much on our own. Their absence was hard on our patients, and on us too.

My heroines, the nurses, pulled me through the year. The first night I was on-call for the medicine service, I admitted three coronary patients, all with typical heart attack symptoms. After hearing their histories and examining them, I wasn't sure what to do next. The head nurse promptly sat down beside me and coached me in writing "nurse's orders"—how often to check pulse, blood pressure and temperature, whether the patient was to be kept at bed rest, what diet and fluids, and what medications were needed for the heart condition, pain, sleep and bowels. Later when I sat down to write their histories, I was so sleepy I could scarcely tell the cases apart, but I had the satisfaction of knowing I had taken good care of my first patients.

We were three women among the twenty-five interns accepted that year. The hospital lodged us conveniently in the nurse's quarters which had quick access to the hospital and was cheap. We received fifty dollars per month with uniforms, laundry, room and board. Kate, my intern roommate, and I shared a bare room with just enough space for two narrow beds. Her cheerful, mischievous outlook lightened the atmosphere. Through the two-foot gap between the beds we could walk to a dresser at one end and a closet at the other end of the room. A phone rested by Kate's bed. Across the hall, Jane, a gynecology resident, had the luxury of a room to herself. Our doors stayed open all the time and Jane kept a coffee machine going. I learned to fight fatigue by drinking her hot, bitter, black coffee.

At seven a.m. interns went to their assigned wards to "draw bloods." The responsible nurse had spent one or two hours the night before or early that morning autoclaving (steam sterilizing) syringes and needles, then sharpening the needles. When we arrived, all the instruments were placed neatly on a cart, with paper slips listing the tests to be done. The ward patients were already sitting up in bed in their bathrobes, with one arm bared for needle puncture. I would walk down the row of beds with the nurse and cart, greet each patient and then draw the amount of blood the nurse indicated. I soon became efficient at puncturing veins and squirting the blood into separate glass tubes containing preservatives.

"Hospital rounds" started at eight a.m., presided by a University Hospital resident. Usually two to three interns and the ward nurse attended. New patients were presented and old patients had their progress appraised. We discussed diagnosis and treatment, then ordered tests and procedures. The resident taught us about the diseases we saw and answered our questions. Once a month a Professor of Medicine came for rounds. We were on our best behavior as we listened attentively for "pearls of wisdom."

Afternoons were reserved for procedures, such as starting intravenous fluids, or doing a "tap." A tap meant removing fluids from some portion of the body, usually chest, abdomen or spinal canal for diagnosis or treatment. Commonly a resident showed us how to do a procedure once, then expected us to do it on our own, "See one, do one, teach one" was the dictum. Inserting a big needle into the body was risky, and at times perspiration poured down my back as I struggled with a difficult procedure. The assisting nurses offered invaluable suggestions, "A little more Doctor, and you're in." "Hold it steady, more fluid is coming out." "Please put the fluid in this test tube for bacterial cultures."

Each open ward held fifteen to twenty patients, and each intern was responsible for a woman's and a man's ward. When patients were acutely or seriously ill, we drew a curtain around their bed, to offer some privacy while we checked on their condition. We were on duty every day and were on "night-call" every third night. "Night-call" included cover of our own wards and those of another intern. When I was on-call, the other intern would find me about four-thirty in the afternoon, to give a run-down of his patients before going off-duty at five. I would be up most of the night attending to his and my patients and admitting new ones. Often on the second evening off-duty, I would still be so tired I would go straight to bed after supper. Only the third off-duty night could I finally stay up and enjoy myself. All too soon the cycle repeated itself.

I remember the night Mr. Allison, a retired teacher, was admitted with chronic leukemia. Although desperately ill, he quietly said, "I know you'll do your best, Doc." Weak and pale, with dark rings around his eyes, he had to sit up to breathe. Fluid rattled in his chest with each breath. Both his liver and spleen were enlarged and his legs swelled with fluid. After repeated phone discussions with the supervising resident, I spent the night trying different ways to remove some of the fluid, but to no avail. He died in the early morning. I was sick at heart.

Patients with diabetic acidosis (very high blood sugars) also kept us up. Every hour we gave varying doses of insulin depending on the concentration of their blood sugars, until the sugar dropped to a safe value. Fortunately, we seldom had more than one such patient at a time.

A heavy-set arthritic man was admitted with non-tender yellowish bumps on his fingers, toes, elbows and knees. Puzzled by these bumps, I withdrew a drop of turbid fluid with a small needle and examined it under the microscope. Tiny sharp-ended crystals filled the field—uric acid crystals. The bumps called tophi were accumulations of these crystals; this man had tophaceous gout. Since routine gout treatment cleared the body of excess uric acid, tophi of such magnitude were rarely seen. I suspected his alcoholism led him to ignore his symptoms until this late stage.

Another "street person" was admitted for generalized pain and dark, red, hemorrhagic (bloody) blotches under the skin. "Gosh, this is scurvy," cried our dermatology resident in disbelief. Scurvy, due to vitamin C deficiency, used to be common among sailors at sea, who did not have fresh citrus fruits to eat. But since people recognized the condition and began drinking orange juice or taking vitamin pills, scurvy was rare—this was another case of neglect and poverty. The patient recovered quickly on large doses of Vitamin C.

During my two months on the medicine service, the main challenges were the common heart, lung and infectious diseases. Streptomycin had just become available for tuberculosis, and sulfa was being used on many infections. Penicillin was still in limited supply because the armed services had priority. We expected these amazing new antibiotics to soon wipe out all infections. Alas, if only that were true.

While on rotation to surgery, I performed two solo procedures with a surgical resident standing by. One procedure was a straightforward appendectomy of a young man, the other, a foot amputation of a diabetic man with a non-healing infected ulcer. I felt so stressed performing these procedures I decided surgery was not for me.

I enjoyed the month in obstetrics under the guidance of Jane, the resident who lived across the hall. I assisted in multiple deliveries, both simple and complicated, and was delighted to deliver two babies myself. This field had its positive side (what joy to produce a baby) but just was not what I wanted to do the rest of my life.

Pediatric service tugged at my heartstrings. I was assigned to deal with babies, not older children. Those tiny crying beings seemed so lost and helpless when ill. Drawing blood for micro tests or starting intravenous fluid on the infants tested my skill and gentleness. And I hated to circumcise the baby boys. I decided my feelings would be too involved to be objective for this specialty.

Rotating from one service to another had its tragi-comical aspects too. A slender, fiftyish, respectable-looking Asian store owner came to the medical outpatient clinic for speech difficulties. A stroke left him able to say only one word, "Damn." It was pitiful to watch him struggle to tell me something, and only come out with an explosive, "Damn!" This being outside my experience, I passed him to neurology outpatient clinic. Imagine our surprise next week when I rotated to the same clinic. I had already read up on his condition, and had to sorrowfully tell him we could not help him recover his speech. Neurologic problems are fascinating to diagnose, but rarely treatable. I wanted to be in a specialty where I could improve the patients' health. After experiencing these different fields, I found I was happiest and did my best work in the field of medicine (in contrast to surgery, pediatrics, etc.). To train further in this field, I would need to take a residency in the specialty of medicine—Internal Medicine.

By a scheduling error, I was given extra months on emergency-ambulance service, so when not on an ambulance call, I toiled long hours in this big city emergency room. The chaos and noise was constant—worse on weekends. I found myself continuously suturing (sewing up) cuts and wounds. Working as fast as I could, I gave short examinations to each entering patient, often including blood tests or x-rays. If I could not take care of them myself, I admitted them to the various hospital floors for further treatment after consulting with the respective intern. I recall a man with a chicken bone wedged in his throat, and another man brought by police from a car accident who walked in but went into shock fifteen minutes later due to internal bleeding from a ruptured spleen. My surgical colleagues took prompt care of them. The pace was so hectic it was hard to relax even when off duty.

What did we do in our time off? Only a few interns or senior nurses had cars, so we were somewhat restricted in activities. My roommate Kate, rotund, black-haired and blue-eyed, was a fun companion on frequent trips for large delicious hamburgers at "King Henry the Eighth" hamburger joint two blocks from the hospital. We took the bus to nearby movie theaters to lose ourselves in the imaginary world on the silver screen. *South Pacific* was one of my favorites. However, my fondest memory was a holiday afternoon and evening spent at the home of a nurse I knew well. Her friendly Scandinavian parents gave us a sumptuous meal. After dinner she played favorite songs on the accordion, while we all joined in the singing. Many years later, the memory of the warm, simple goodness of these Scandinavians may have drawn me back to Minnesota.

This whirlwind year, full of surprises, learning and exhaustion, had stretched my thinking, feeling and strength. It seemed I had seen every problem in medicine, and learned to handle many of them. I had helped a few people, but for others I could only standby and comfort; there were limitations to what a physician could do. Now I was ready to enter three years of residency training in my chosen specialty of Internal Medicine. It was to be one of the most wonderful periods in my life.

Chapter 9

ROCHESTER, MN:
THE WORLD OF MAYO 1951-55

The acceptance telegram seemed to burn in my white uniform pocket. For two days I fingered it several times a day, not knowing what to do. I dared not believe an Asian immigrant woman had actually been accepted for physician training by the world famous Mayo Clinic. I had applied there on a long shot, along with other applications, not expecting anything. Now this telegram read, "You are accepted for an Internal Medicine residency program commencing Jan. 1, 1951." To complicate matters, I had already accepted a position at Baylor College of Medicine, Houston, Texas. Could I in good conscience withdraw? I phoned the Professor of Medicine at Baylor. His magnanimous reply was, "How wonderful for you. You are hereby released from your acceptance. Our best wishes!"

On a clear, cold day on December 28, 1950, I moved to Rochester, Minnesota, a town of thirty-two thousand then, just ninety miles south of Minneapolis. The Mayo Clinic stood in the midst of rolling hills of cornfields, covered with two inches of snow. A local business woman rented me a comfortable room in her two-story home within walking distance of the two places where I was to work—the Mayo Clinic and St. Marys Hospital. My hundred-fifty dollar monthly salary amply covered the fifty dollar rent.

Tingling with awe and anticipation, on January first, I climbed a few steps and passed through the fifteen-foot tall, intricately carved bronze doors into the elegant Italianate Plummer Building which housed the Mayo Clinic. Since I had previously only worked in dull, plain cement buildings, this beautiful place filled me with wonder. A smiling receptionist pointed along a red-blue-tan marble floor to a bank of elevators. Another young woman took me up to my first assignment, the Cardiology section on the ninth floor.

A white-uniformed desk supervisor approached me with a friendly, "Good morning, Dr. Ling. Welcome. I've been asked to introduce you to our set-up."

Timidly I asked, "May I interrupt with questions?"

"Of course, please do. The Mayo brothers, Dr. Will and Dr. Charlie, organized this fifteen-story building solely for outpatient care. In doing this, they created the country's first private group practice. Today, about three hundred full-time staff physicians, who we call "consultants," and a large number of young residents-in-training, like you, treat about four hundred patients a day. Our staff of administrators, desk persons, secretaries, dietitians, social workers, librarians and translators are here to help you every way we can."

I responded, "Yes, the famous brothers were wonderful surgeons. I believe they died about ten years ago. Didn't doctors come from all over the world to observe their surgeries?"

"Right. Even today their legacy of first class surgery still draws many visiting physicians."

She continued, "For a long time our practice has been to require all patients, medical or surgical (except the desperately ill), to first pass a preliminary medical evaluation in this Outpatient Clinic."

As we walked down the hall, she pointed to the arrangements saying, "Floors 4 to 11 are pretty much like this one. In this large center patient lobby, half the upholstered chairs face the North desk, half face the South desk. Patients wait here until they are called by attendants, commonly called 'desk girls,' who guide them to examining rooms along the north or south corridors."

Opening the door of a windowed examining room, she continued, "Here there is a sofa for the patient, a doctor's desk and an examining table next to a wash basin. Such things as thermometers, tongue blades, alcohol swabs and culture tubes are stored in this cupboard over the basin, while towels and gowns are kept in these drawers under the examining table."

She pointed to a curtained niche next to the door, "The patients change here." I noticed height-weight scales standing nearby, and blood pressure cuff and other equipment hanging on the wall next to the examining table. She added with a smile, "You'll notice there is a brass name tag on the door with the name of a consultant staff physician. They can put personal books on the shelves above the desk, hang diplomas on the wall, or use the room any way they like, but when they are out, any other doctor can use the room to see patients. This room sharing not only makes good use of space, but avoids room ownership problems."

"What are those lights for?" I asked, pointing to a vertical row of colored lights alongside the door outside each room.

"When a patient is inside, a white light goes on. Each doctor entering the room turns on his or her own light pattern—yours will be yellow and green. We, at the Desk, can tell at a glance what is happening inside each room. If another doctor or desk attendant wishes to talk to you, they will page you so you can phone back."

"Do these long bins in your Desk area hold medical records?" I asked, pointing to them.

"Yes, the entire patients' history is in their medical records. It follows them to each appointment. For example, a man with heart failure sees a cardiologist, but if he has cataracts he then sees an ophthalmologist. If he suffers urinary problems he also sees an urologist. Since the specialists work on different floors, they coordinate their work using these integrated records. Dr. Henry Plummer, the designer of this building, devised a conveyer and pneumatic tube system to speedily carry records to different floors."

The orientation finished, she took me to meet Dr. Thomas Dry, my first supervising consultant. A tall, quick-moving man, he spoke in clipped words with a hint of a South African accent.

"Dr. Ling, you will see at least three patients each morning. After a careful history and physical exam, please present each case to me. I may go in and check some of your findings. We will formulate a diagnosis together and decide on appropriate tests. Understood?"

"Yes, very clear."

"I will then take over the case. You may come in to observe our discussion over test results. After reviewing the results, I will offer the patient my diagnosis and outline a treatment plan. If you have questions we will talk about them later, but not in front of the patient. After patient dismissal, I will dictate a summary to the referring physician. When it is typed, you get a final review of the case. Any questions?"

"No, Doctor." Although I didn't have questions then, I certainly had many later.

Most of the difficult cases sent to the Clinic specialists had complicated histories. The work-ups took so much time I barely finished three patients each morning. Dr. Dry was an authority on congestive heart failure and heart valve defects. These problems dominated Cardiology at the time. Always courteous, he carefully explained his opinions and answered each patient's questions. I tried hard to pattern myself after him.

After the hectic internship at the Minneapolis City hospital, the quiet dignity of the Mayo Clinic seemed like a religious retreat. We medical residents were really apprentices to the specialists who taught and monitored us. Because of Mayo's emphasis on outpatient care, we first spent two years "on the floors" of the Clinic, then finished the third year in the hospitals, caring for even sicker patients.

The founding Mayo brothers had devised an outstanding residency training program. I rotated through required medical subspecialty sections, but also had a wide choice of other sections. I chose to train in subspecialties of Cardiology (heart), Rheumatology (joints) and Endocrinology (hormones[13]) and added time in other sections of Neuro-psychiatry and Obstetrics-gynecology. Most rotations lasted three months. I spent my laboratory time in Pathology examining tissues under the microscope. My hospital rotation followed similar choices.

The consultant doctors constantly challenged us residents to diagnose and suggest treatments for complex cases. We participated in weekly seminars and monthly staff meetings, and spent spare time studying in the medical library or working in the laboratories. Working with giants in their fields was a heady experience! These staff members had written numerous papers and had become sought-after speakers at national conferences. Since difficult cases were often referred to Mayo, it gave us the opportunity to see a large number of rare medical conditions.

---

[13]   Hormones: tiny amounts of essential substances that profoundly affect the whole body. They are produced by a gland and secreted into the blood stream. Each hormone, such as cortisone, thyroid hormone or insulin, has very specific effects.

After a month at Mayo, we all knew of our Nobel Prize winner of 1950, Dr. Philip Hench, a rheumatologist. His use of recently discovered cortisone[14] hormone to treat rheumatoid arthritis led to its widespread use in many illnesses. I was so intrigued by his discovery, I requested rotation to Rheumatology in my first year. Dr. Hench was a tall man with a loud voice. His nasal speech, due to a cleft palate, did not deter him. Wherever he was, his voice dominated the room. He loved to tell how during World War II, he outwitted malingering soldiers who tried using back pain to obtain sick leave. After each story he would roar with laughter. I also felt sympathy for him when he, a migraine sufferer, periodically stomped down the corridor announcing loudly, "I'm going home. I have an awful headache." He started the Rheumatology section at Mayo, and helped to put this new subspecialty on the national scene. I suspect his influence was important in my own decision to later specialize in Rheumatology.

Dr. Edward Rynearson, another consultant I delighted in, made us all laugh. A tall commanding presence, he would arrive on the floor announcing to the stressed young desk attendants, "Be good to me, girls. I've had a tough time. This is 'Be Kind to Rynearson Day!'" I could feel the tension ease as they burst into laughter. An endocrinologist, he saw many patients with weight problems. He told us of one woman who said, "But Dr. Rynearson, I eat like a bird." "Yes," he replied, "like a vulture." How he got away with such answers I don't know, but his patients adored him. A dahlia grower, he presented me one

---

14 Cortisone: a potent hormone produced by the adrenal glands—a small gland on top of each kidney—that works on the body's immune system. While important in treating many conditions, it has unpleasant side effects.

day with a six-inch wide pink dahlia. "For you, Dr. Ling," he said. I was enchanted.

Endocrinology was largely caring for thyroid[15] diseases and diabetes mellitus[16]. Accompanying Dr. Rynearson on hospital rounds meant checking on patients recovering from thyroid operations—many for removal of benign goiters, prevalent in the Midwest from drinking iodine-deficient water. After rounds, over coffee and rolls at a nearby cafe, he would teach us about various thyroid diseases.

I will never forget his profound lesson in patient care. Betsy was a well-liked thirty-year old dietitian with severe diabetes. In spite of good care of her own diabetes, she developed serious complications—first vision deterioration, then kidney failure. Finally, multiple emboli (blood clots in arteries) to her brain left her unconscious and surviving only on intravenous fluids. When another embolus blocked a major leg artery, amputation would have been the only recourse. Dr. Rynearson gathered her family, whom he knew well, by her bedside to discuss what should be done for Betsy. They all agreed it would be best to let her go. Then Dr. Rynearson pulled out her intravenous tubing. Later, having never regained consciousness, while her family held her hands, she quietly died. There is a point of no return for a patient when a good physician must have the courage to let nature take its course.

---

[15] Thyroid: a gland that sits at the base of the neck and produces thyroid hormone. This hormone regulates the body's mental and physical speed.

[16] Diabetes mellitus: a disease from lack of the hormone insulin. Insulin is produced by the pancreas gland that lies in the middle of the body, behind the stomach.

Dr. Harry Lee Parker was a gruff neurologist from Ireland. Although a big bear of a man with thick glasses and a drooping mustache, he was gentle with his patients. While I was working in Neurology, I would answer my page to hear his deep voice, "Ling, come here." He would then introduce me to a patient with some abnormal nerve disorder.

One time, he said, "Examine his right hand and wrist where he has pain, numbness and tingling. What nerve innervates the palm side of the first three fingers?" I answered, "The median nerve." "Right," he said, then told me an abnormal protein had been deposited at the man's wrist, blocking this nerve function. Dr. Parker was a born teacher, making even the discussion of common migraine headaches a fascinating subject. Since the nervous system controls the whole body, almost every disease influences this system in some way, and vice versa. He helped me to understand this important field. With the deep respect in which we held our teachers, I sometimes called at his home on weekends. His wife served tea while he held forth on Neurology and Ireland. I thought of him often when I later practiced medicine in Ireland.

I also recall Dr. Adelaide Johnson, a brilliant child psychiatrist. She was one of three women consultants then on staff. During my Psychiatry rotation, I attended her seminars. Elegant in expensive suits, she held court among the residents analyzing new cases. I was always afraid she would call on me, for she could sharply cut a person down for the wrong answer. In one seminar, she presented the hypothesis that a misbehaving child in a family of well-behaved siblings might be acting out forbidden wishes of a parent. She described a small boy who played truant to attend ball games, and was caught stealing several hundred dollars worth of sports equipment. She discovered the father had secretly wanted to do these things but never dared, and was covertly encouraging the boy. I was impressed with her shrewd interpretation.

Although Mayo was male-oriented, I did not feel strange to be one of a dozen women among over a hundred new residents. The same gender ratio had existed in medical school. I expected to work in man's world, and I liked their way of analyzing problems to find solutions. A clinician at heart, I felt comfortable with Mayo's priorities: patient care, education and research.

Mayo male physicians' early awareness of the female invasion of their stronghold happened at a dinner to welcome new residents. For some reason I was the only woman sitting with a group of men. After a pleasant dinner, the consultant proceeded to tell some off-color jokes. Suddenly he stopped, and turning red-faced to me, he stammered, "I apologize, Dr. Ling, I'm not used to the presence of ladies at these gatherings." Throughout my years at Mayo, I can candidly say I have always been courteously treated with complete equality in all dealings with colleagues and staff.

Mayo had accepted only single men and women in their residency program, presumably because marriage might distract them from their studies. Although this rule had been relaxed by 1951, the majority of residents were still single. The few married couples usually lived in Quonset huts built by the Clinic during World War II. We use to call the area "fertile valley" due to the many pregnancies and children.

Most of the women residents chose Internal Medicine, but a few hardy souls each chose Gynecology, Pediatrics, Ophthalmology, Orthopedic surgery, Neurology and Psychiatry. All but two of us were single. Since we worked in different areas of the Clinic or hospital, we only met intermittently, usually one-on-one for meals. I knew them all, but my two special friends were Madeline Wong in Gynecology and Joan Brady in Pediatrics. Madeline was a Chinese woman from Vancouver, Canada. Barely five feet tall, slender, quiet and unassuming, she was busy training in her field. I saw her mainly in her apartment, where we enjoyed cooking and eating Chinese food together. My housemate Joan was a bespectacled, plump, voluble second-generation Irish American. We shared many suppers in local restaurants where she regaled me with stories about her physician father's general practice and her life in New York City.

We residents were often invited to consultants' homes on holidays such as Thanksgiving. I loved getting better acquainted with them and their families in these informal settings. In my second year I began attending larger parties given by Dr. Maurice Barry, a psychiatrist. He and his wife, Shirley, were wonderful hosts for lonely young people. One met "everyone" at these parties lasting into the small morning hours. They had a large library of interesting books, plenty of jazz to listen and dance to, and a long table laden with delicious food. Resident dances also took place in a roomy barn at Mayowood, the former farm estate of Dr. Charles Mayo. I remember one autumn party where shocks of corn were scattered around the barn. We all dressed in "country clothes"—plaid shirts and jeans for men, and cotton frocks with wide skirts for women. Beer flowed freely as we danced into the night.

Toward the end of my second year I rotated to hospital Psychiatry where I met Dr. Peter Beckett, a senior resident. I immediately liked this cheerful, fun-loving young man from Dublin, Ireland. He was barely taller than I was at five-feet-five, with the typical Irish pink complexion and bright blue eyes. His innocent boyish look, engaging smile, gentle humor and easy ways made many friends. As he began to teach me psychiatry, I discovered under his charming exterior was a curious wide-open mind, interested in everything. He also started teaching me to drive his old, stick-shift, two-seater Ford. Loving outdoors and picnics, he asked me to pack bread, cheese and fruit for trips to the surrounding countryside. We especially enjoyed walking along the Mississippi River banks on the Minnesota side, or crossing the river to the Wisconsin side, to climb to the top of the bluffs in Trempealeau Park and look down on the river as we picnicked.

Later he accompanied me to the Barry parties, or took me to meet his married Irish doctor friends in the Quonset huts. Growing ever closer over the year, we were married on January 11, 1954 on a brisk, cold but sunny day at the local Methodist church. The snow was knee-high and we were bundled in warm coats when outdoors. Attending were my parents, sister, brother and Mrs. Dunn, but Peter's siblings and mother could not make the long trip from Ireland. We had trouble choosing the few from among our many friends, colleagues and teachers who could fit into the small church and reception hall. Our best man was a Psychiatry resident from Munich, and the maid-of-honor was my friend, Joan Brady. My dear Peter, in his borrowed blue suit, wore a perpetual smile, telling everyone, "This is the happiest day of my life."

A year later, we both became U.S. citizens in a solemn courtroom proceeding. Because of prohibitive immigration laws, this had taken me seven years. A Minnesota Congress Representative, a prior missionary to China, came to my rescue by, "extracting my papers from the bottom of the pile to put them on top." Additional helpful letters from the Mayo Clinic were decisive in moving my case forward. To renounce citizenship of one's country of birth is a profound step, but Peter and I had decided to make a life together in America.

In the summer of 1955, we completed our time at Mayo. We were both recommended for consultancy, but the Clinic did not permit both husband and wife to be on staff, so we elected to take up posts in Michigan.

Nothing could compare with those four Rochester years. I had been exposed to the best minds in medicine, observed the finest standards of medical care and completed my training as a specialist in Internal Medicine, all the while enjoying every moment. Moreover, I had gained a husband and become an American citizen.

Chapter 10

DETROIT:

THE MATURING YEARS 1955-69

On a sweltering day in July 1955 we arrived in Detroit—the "motor city" of America on the Great Lakes. After considering all of Peter's job options, we had selected the assistant directorship of the brand new Lafayette Clinic, a 145-bed psychiatric research and training hospital under the Michigan Department of Mental Health. Under the dynamic leadership of Dr. J. Gottlieb, Peter would supervise the training of psychiatrists for the state of Michigan, and lead a serious research program.

This program followed the thesis that young people with schizophrenia had a biochemical brain defect. Finding a cause for this mental illness would be an exciting breakthrough in Psychiatry. To study such a mechanism, an outstanding biochemist had been recruited, a powerful computer installed and many small experimental animals collected. One day Peter came home laughing. "As you know, the engineers are struggling to install air-conditioning in our new building. While we doctors sweltered in our offices dripping with sweat, the engineers directed most of the cool air to the computer and animal rooms. We learned just how important we are."

To start our married life together, Peter and I had to make some important decisions. We considered being a biracial couple quite special. Peter said, "Didn't we come halfway across the world to meet and marry?" After acknowledging the possibility of discrimination toward us or our children, we decided to face problems together as they arose.

I struggled with conflicting desires before deciding to postpone full-time medical practice to start raising a family. I wanted Peter's career to come first—he would be head of the family. Peter wanted our marriage to be teamwork, where both of us had equal rights and responsibilities. We concluded he would be the major breadwinner, while I would be the main family manager.

Another issue was Peter's draft status as a new U.S. citizen. To our relief we discovered his two years in the British Army Medical Corp fulfilled his U.S. service requirement. We could now make definite plans for our future.

We bought a one-story house in an eastern suburb of Detroit, with its own small park on adjacent Lake St. Clair. I later learned an Asian would not have been admitted into this suburb except that I had married Peter, a Caucasian. However, once settled in our cozy little house, we lived happily for over a decade among helpful, friendly neighbors.

I soon started clinical teaching at Wayne State Medical School, and also established a part-time medical practice at Henry Ford Hospital. With jobs and home secure, Peter and I could finally develop a meaningful marriage relationship.

Who was this young man? He would enter a room with a bounce, often hand in pocket, his bright eyes quickly scanning around and a slight smile on his lips. Peter's sunny personality seemed to light up the room; people would turn toward him in welcome. He was a cheerful, easy-going man with simple tastes. Encountering a difficulty, he would offer a joke or a solution and then pass on. I cannot recall a single time he was rude or really angry. A warm, loving helpmate, he was always ready to support and comfort me. Like his name, "Peter the rock," he was completely trustworthy and dependable. I learned he kept every promise, no matter how difficult. Of his amazing resourcefulness, I used to say jokingly, "Peter, if I needed a companion to be marooned with on a desert island, I would choose you. I'm sure you would find food and shelter, and know how to hail a passing ship!"

My, I thought, I was no longer alone, but had someone to share all joys and sorrows. How wonderful! I had been self-sufficient alone, but with Peter at my side, I felt able to face any adversity.

Perhaps Peter's most important gift to me was a new optimism toward life. I had grown up believing life was a valley of tears that one had to get through as best one could. Peter said, "Nonsense, don't believe that. Life is a great adventure, a game to play to win." Gradually, his zest for life, his looking forward to every challenge, his planning ahead and getting things done, led me to believe in his viewpoint. He thought I took things too seriously and worked too hard. He used to say, "I wish you would just relax. Sit down and put your feet up. Let me take care of things."

Peter loved the outdoors, something completely new to me. No one in my family bothered to look at a blade of grass; happenings in nature simply did not register. To help me see and appreciate such natural beauty, Peter introduced me to various outdoor activities. He almost immediately purchased a small, twin-hulled catamaran to sail on Lake St. Clair. Our local park had picnic grounds, a swimming pool and most importantly a boat dock. Flying over the water in our small craft with Peter at the helm was exhilarating; my sole task was to pull the jib rope at his command. As his work became more stressful, he often stopped to sail for an hour in the evening before coming home relaxed and cheerful for supper. In summer, his Saturdays were spent sailboat racing with his friends as a member of the Lake St. Clair sailing fraternity.

On Sundays we drove into the countryside "to see what nature was doing," as we explored rural roads and small farm areas. An avid bird-watcher with excellent distant vision, Peter would suddenly stop the car, whip out his binoculars and exclaim, "See the redwing? See the scarlet patches on his wings?" He filled Peterson's bird book with entries of dates and comments on what he saw. Being near-sighted I never saw the birds before they flew away, but I learned to wonder at the flying creatures and to listen to their songs. Picnics were standard at the outings; I could pack a quick lunch at a moment's notice. It was such fun to lean back and let Peter lead wherever he wanted.

My introduction to the outdoors included our first trip to Ireland, soon after marriage, when Peter took me to meet his mother and sister. Ann, his sister, met us at the Dublin airport. She was a cheerful, quick-moving young woman, strongly resembling Peter. She had the same pink skin, blue eyes and gray hair. We drove to the family home in Greystones, just south of Dublin. As we turned into the gate, there was my mother-in-law, a heavy-set woman with snow-white hair, leaning on a cane. Her beaming smile instantly made me feel welcome. Directly after a brief get-acquainted lunch, she showed us her garden—the center of her love and labor. Its beauty took my breath away!

A six-foot hedge of golden gorse surrounded this two-acre garden; the shrub's prickly surface kept out the cows of the neighboring farmer. Below it was a four-foot sloping bank on which she had planted delphiniums, lupines, oriental poppies, foxglove, pansies, lamb's ear, silver pennies, bleeding hearts, lavender and more. She grouped six to twelve plants of a kind to form solid masses of color. Since she favored soft colors, I saw patches of white, blue, pink, mauve, light yellow and gray, with only small dabs of orange or red. A weeping willow tree shaded a small pond in the center. In a corner was a bed of a dozen varieties of roses, and behind them two rows of raspberry bushes. A large bed of compost fed the entire garden. The watering came from the wet skies above. Ma Beckett was already a self-taught painter, and in this garden she had created a stunning live painting. I have never seen a garden to match it, and I spent every spare minute sitting outdoors drinking in its beauty.

She said, "My dear, you must start a garden." This was a brand new idea, but after seeing her garden, I agreed. On return to Detroit, I began planting flowers around our house. The more I gardened, the more I loved it. With new awareness, I now often gaze at the sky, note the weather, observe the beauty and changes of trees and flowers, and look forward to each new season, enjoying the cycle of life.

Peter had a good ear and a deep appreciation of classical music. Once a month he would come home with a new record to play during dinner. There always seemed to be music in the background whenever he relaxed. I learned to listen and to enjoy evening concerts with him. During his Rochester days Peter had discovered jazz; a favorite record was Louis Armstrong playing his trumpet and singing *I'm So Black and Blue*. When the Beatles took the country by storm, we also listened with curiosity and interest to their rendition of *Lucy in the Sky with Diamonds*.

With pride I could say I developed a creative art form myself—cooking. When I was first married I didn't know how to cook, even burning the breakfast toast. In dismay I phoned my mother, an excellent cook, for some simple recipes. Within a week a dozen carefully written recipes arrived. This took a real effort for Mother, who cooked by instinct and taste. I gratefully followed her recipes, until I could place tasty dishes in front of Peter. His appreciative response had me scanning many cookbooks to begin producing mouth-watering Chinese, American, Italian and French dishes. I must have inherited some of Mother's culinary instincts. With America's cornucopia of the world's finest raw ingredients, how could I lose? My cooking was a decided asset when I put on picnics for Peter's psychiatric residents or dinners for our physician friends. Becoming known as a good hostess pleased me immensely.

And so the happy days slipped by. I often pinched myself to be sure they were real.

We began to plan a family. After a year of infertility studies, we had to choose either not to have children or to adopt. There were no alternatives then. We wanted the fulfillment of having children. We had great hopes of passing on what we had learned of hope, tolerance and truth. We searched for an Asian-Caucasian boy who would look like one of our own. During the frustrating adoption procedure, I began to voice a concern. "Peter, what if the adopted child doesn't turn out well?" Peter replied, "You mustn't think that way. We couldn't guarantee a child of our own would turn out well. Besides, we can first examine the child before we adopt him."

A year later we were offered a healthy, plump, alert and smiling baby boy, just six months old. We immediately wanted him. Baby Paul came to live with us, becoming our precious son. Our family was finally complete. When Peter stressed the crucial importance of a child's first five developmental years, I thought, who could take care of him better than I could? I decided to continue my weekly medical school teaching, but forego practicing medicine. I would knuckle down to be a full-time mother and wife. Thus started five serene, fulfilling years.

Being a physician didn't help me much in raising a baby. I could not have done it without Dr. Spock's baby care book or the advice from friends with children. The arousal of strong, protective maternal instinct surprised me. Certainly the care and nurture of my own child was completely different from taking care of someone else's child.

As Baby Paul grew, I relived the wonder of a child discovering the world around him. He viewed the night sky and stars with wonder. "Mama, stars." He loved the blinking Christmas tree lights. "Mama, light." Organ music heralded the ice cream man's cart, bringing him and the neighbor children running. "Ice cream, Mama." A quick learner, he could name colors and read simple Dr. Seuss books by the time he was three. Attending a nearby preschool center and playing with neighboring little ones helped him learn to get along with other children. With enthusiasm, I took him to children's concerts, the local public library and the park playground. Motherhood turned out to be an expanding, softening, emotional experience, quite beyond my expectations.

Peter took special delight in spending time with our son on evenings and weekends. During weekend outings, little Paul loved to play hide-and-seek with his father in the woods. On the catamaran, he was tethered to the mast wearing his life jacket. How he laughed with glee to feel the wind and spray wash over him. He learned to swim and become a good little sailor.

As he grew older, Peter took us on camping trips, teaching Paul how to put up a tent, light a fire and manage camp food. He also taught him to ride a bicycle and do repairs on it. I was delighted to see father and son talking, laughing and doing things together. Our small son looked up to his father as they developed a strong comradeship.

Because his birthday was on December 31st, Paul was in the awkward position of being too old for one school class and too young for the other. Contrary to the teacher's opinion, Peter put him with the younger children because he felt an only child needed time to mature emotionally. As a result, Paul often found schoolwork unchallenging. We tried to stimulate his interests by taking him with us on trips—to Dublin, London, Copenhagen, Jamaica, Hawaii and Washington D.C. We watched his development with pride and satisfaction.

When Paul turned six, I returned to practicing medicine. The first post offered me at the Henry Ford Hospital was in the new medical subspecialty of Oncology. Oncology patients had cancer spread beyond surgical removal. In those early days of chemotherapy, these people became deathly sick on the treatment and their improvement was transient. While the practice had many depressing aspects, I do recall some uplifting cases. One was an elderly Greek woman with breast cancer who was rapidly going downhill in spite of treatment. She wanted desperately to live long enough to take part in her youngest son's wedding. Promising to help, I filled her full of medicines to temporarily make her feel better. At her insistence I attended the wedding. It was a traditional elaborate Greek wedding, a beautiful, heart-warming event filled with dancing, singing, plenty of whisky and delicious food. Most of the Greek community in Detroit attended. She was the queen of the evening. We both loved every minute of it.

Finally, I decided to switch to Rheumatology. I was at my best dealing with patients directly, listening to their stories and doing a careful physical examination to make the diagnosis and to guide treatment, all without many laboratory tests. This specialty would be dealing with chronic conditions, such as gout, rheumatoid arthritis and osteoarthritis. I felt I could help these people live a fairly normal life span by offering ways to cope with their disabilities. This was a wise choice when I later practiced in a country where sophisticated laboratory tests were unavailable.

Over the ensuing years, I watched in proud amazement as Peter developed various abilities. Initially a good psychiatrist, he became an outstanding teacher, loved and admired by the young residents. An effective administrator, his door was always open to others; he settled several sensitive racial conflicts between black and white employees. As a researcher he worked hard on the schizophrenia research project. Although they were unable to discover the specific biochemical defect in this disease, his numerous papers on their work earned him a national reputation. This led to his appointment to the national Psychiatric Board of Examiners to certify doctors in the specialty of Psychiatry. He co-authored two psychiatry teaching manuals. His new systematic, question-and-answer writing method was popular among the young doctors. His interest in young people also led him to organize one of the first hospital units for treating adolescents, and to write a well-received monograph *Adolescents Out of Step: Their Treatment in a Psychiatric Hospital*. One of his close colleagues confided to me, "I think Peter's blossoming is due to his stable happy marriage." I thought it a wonderful compliment.

Peter and I went on numerous interesting professional meeting trips together, followed by side trips. After an international psychiatric meeting in Geneva, Switzerland, we rented a car and drove south across the Alps to Genoa, then to Paris. In Paris I met for the only time, my famous writer cousin, Samuel Beckett. A tall, quiet, thoughtful man, he seemed bewildered yet pleased with his sudden success. At a restaurant, while he was introducing me to *escargot,* Frenchmen kept coming up to congratulate him upon his recent Nobel Prize. He told us, with amusement, his books had accumulated large sums of money behind the Iron Curtain. Since he was not allowed to take any of it out, he would periodically travel to these communist countries for wild spending sprees with friends. When asked the message in his famous play *Waiting for Godot,* he replied, "No message. Persons must find their own message based on their life experiences."

After Paul was five we took him on most of our trips. He found the seashore in Maui, Hawaii a perfect paradise. Rome, with its exquisite art in St. Peter's Cathedral and the Sistine Chapel, and its delicious cuisine, was one of Peter's favorite places. I loved both places too. When Peter was exchange professor in Jamaica for three months, he studied the influence of voodoo on medical cases. He concluded its success could be due to a placebo effect—the people's strong belief in the witch doctor's claims helped to make them come true. Peter mused, "If I give a big, red, dotted pill to a patient and tell him it would make him well, maybe he would believe me enough to get well."

Life however, never remains smooth for long. Mother suffered a stroke while Christmas shopping with Father, and died a few hours later. She had been so much a part of my life as supporter, role model and loving presence, I wasn't sure at first if I could go on without her. I need not have worried, for somehow, even now, I feel her still with me, cheering me on.

During the Cuban missile crisis, Peter was at a meeting in Washington D.C. I could hear the fear in his voice when he phoned to warn he might not be able to get home if war developed. Luckily, we averted war. Our continued fear of nuclear war prompted us to start building a bomb shelter in our basement. We were particularly anxious to assure Paul's survival to carry on the human race. I can laugh at it now, but we were quite serious then.

The social turmoil of the 1960s greatly disturbed us. Marijuana intruded in our local schools so seriously, we feared for our son. The Detroit race riot necessitated calling in the National Guards for control. Since the Lafayette Clinic was downtown near the riot area, Peter had to arrange police escorts for his employees to get to work. He himself was in danger during his daily commute from the suburbs. The big "DOCTOR" sign he put on the roof of his car may have guarded him.

Shortly afterward, President Kennedy, his brother and the Rev. Martin Luther King Jr. were assassinated. We began thinking of moving elsewhere. In his middle forties, Peter declared, "If we don't move now, we never will." He did not want to become the Director of the clinic, whose main job was to pry money from the state legislature. After investigating several proffered alternatives, a job in Ireland won his heart.

The dozen years in Detroit may seem uneventful, but this relaxed period may have been our happiest time together. We had the peace of mind to develop in our professions, and to become a happy, healthy family.

Our new maturity was about to be tested in new and different ways.

Chapter 11

IRELAND:

SWEET AND BITTER YEARS 1969-76

I can still see the glowing pleasure on Peter's face as he read the invitation to form a psychiatric department at his alma mater, the medical school of Trinity College, Dublin University. I felt sure he was thinking, "How can I refuse my own school?"

This idea of moving to Ireland was at first hard for me to accept.

"But Peter," I said, "you are established here. Do you really want to give up such excellent prospects? You would take a big salary cut and give up your pension. Besides, what could I do there? And you know how I dislike that cold damp weather."

"Don't worry, my salary will be adequate to live comfortably. Things are much cheaper there. With your qualifications, you should easily find satisfying medical work. They will be lucky to have you. I can't change the weather, but I promise you we will live in a house with central heating."

He continued, "It's not fair to live so well here, and give nothing back to the home country." He clinched the matter by reminding me, "You wanted to go back to help China, but the Communist take-over stopped you. Why shouldn't we go back to my country, where I could actually do something worthwhile? Anyway, we can come back after about five years. Then I could consult or teach psychiatry and you could practice medicine here again."

With some hesitation I eventually agreed.

In America, Peter was known as a good psychiatrist, one among many, but in tiny Ireland, where the title of Professor produces awe, he immediately had enormous prestige and importance. He was welcomed as a successful native son who chose to return, and he enthusiastically applied his America experience to his new job. He started by teaching medical students how to do a good psychiatric interview. Since there was no biochemical test for mental illnesses and a physical examination was rarely helpful, a good psychiatric interview was the key to making an accurate diagnosis. He devised the novel teaching method of videotaping each student's one-on-one patient interview. Later he replayed it for the whole class to watch and critique. I don't believe any student slept through that class. They also used his popular student teaching manuals.

Next, he proceeded to organize a three-year psychiatric resident training program open to all graduates of medical schools in the Irish Republic. His colleagues warned of social, political and religious impediments, and greeted his projects with the well-worn phrase, "not in my lifetime." Peter thanked them for their concerns, then quietly proceeded to institute his changes, often succeeding before anyone had time to object. The residency program was in place by his third year in Ireland. An effective, practical person, he had the rare ability to make changes without antagonizing others. Furthermore, his colleagues grew to trust him as an outsider without entrenched interests or personal aggrandizement.

His new Psychiatry Department managed hospital units treating mental illness. When he saw how serious alcoholism was in Ireland, he embarked on research to understand and help cope with this problem. He observed two types of alcoholics: one, usually found among the Mediterranean population who drank wine all day and although slightly high could work adequately; the other, usually found among the Irish who after one drink, completely lost control. He was also surprised to observe a high incidence of alcoholic dementia in Ireland, while in American alcoholic liver cirrhosis was more common. Peter began epidemiological studies on alcoholism in various parts of Ireland. He also undertook studies on the effects of alcohol on experimental rats, and we often teased him about his "drunken rats."

Three years later, when the Dean of the Medical School at Trinity retired, Peter was quickly elected to take his place. He hoped this new position would give him the authority to make major improvements in the medical school.

I objected, "No, you shouldn't take on two full-time jobs."

But he replied, "I will leave the day-to-day department work to my three able assistant psychiatrists. I'll be on call and regularly meet with them once a week. Of course, I'll also continue my lectures. Don't worry, if it's too much, I promise I will give up one of the jobs." Accordingly, he spent most of his time busy at the Dean's office with a newly hired administrative assistant.

How did Paul and I fare during this time? After Paul's unsatisfactory year at a local school, we transferred our eleven-year-old to a private boy's boarding school, St. Columba. Its high academic standards were modeled after the English schools. Although I thought him too young to live away from home, Peter convinced me this was the way boys in the British Isles were raised. He himself had gone to such a school. I was pleased to see how well Paul settled in and made good friends, but I missed him.

We bought a two-story house with central heating in a new suburb just north of Dublin. Sutton is located at the neck of the Howth peninsula. My first task was to tackle the wide cracks between the wooden floorboards in the living/dining room.

"It's the central heating, mum," said the floor man shaking his head. "It does dreadful things, like making the boards shrink. There's nothing to do, I'm afraid." Undaunted, I covered the floors with cork squares, like those at the Mayo Clinic, and they worked well.

Next, I ordered wall-to-wall carpets for the upstairs study and bedrooms. I dashed home at the appointed hour, but the carpet man didn't come. The next day I called him.

"Och, I'm sorry, mum. My ma suddenly took sick and I had to put her in hospital. Why didn't I call? Well, I was that worried I forgot." When he came the following week, I stood over him until he finished laying all the carpets.

Later, I booked a salesman of a large downtown department store to measure for kitchen cupboards and shelves. When he failed to show up, I called to ask why. He said, "Mum, I'm terrible sorry, but I had to take my ma to the hospital as she came down with the pneumonia, and I plum forgot about meeting you." I complained to his supervisor, who said, "Paddy was probably getting over a hangover since he didn't come to work that day. I'll see that he gets to your place tomorrow for sure, else he'll get the sack." He came, and I got my kitchen cupboards and shelves.

I asked the plumber why my kitchen faucets were labeled "H" for cold water and "C" for hot water. He answered with a knowing smile, "Well now, the man probably had a bit of the drink when he connected them, mum."

We ordered three flowering apple trees with pink blossoms for the garden. The nurseryman promised he had just the trees, and he would personally bring a companion to plant them the following week. Five phone calls and a month later the trees were planted. They turned out to be pear trees bearing white blossoms. And so it went. I did find reliable workers, but charming rascals were common. Amusing yet frustrating, every activity took twice the time and effort it would have taken in America.

Peter had warned me Ireland was a wonderful place to grow up and retire, but a terrible place to work. It is a tiny sparsely populated island, confined by the Atlantic Ocean on one side and England on the other. A poor country with few good jobs, it could only urge its most energetic and talented to emigrate. Peter had worried I might feel claustrophobic in such a small country, and find "everything fifty years behind." I felt I could accommodate to these conditions, but was not prepared for the obstacles to my practicing medicine. In spite of my advanced American specialist qualifications, the medical authorities insisted I pass the Irish medical licensing examinations. It took a year and a half to plow through the red tape and paperwork to pass the exams. I was then allowed to teach at the medical school, run the outpatient Rheumatic clinic and take care of hospital rheumatic inpatients, but only under the supervision of the Professor of Medicine, and without pay. Remembering why we were there, I accepted. At least I would see Irish medicine from the inside.

A pleasant surprise was the discovery of the "Anglo-Irish" community. Peter was a part of this small Protestant minority, which comprised only one or two percent of the predominantly Catholic population. These Anglo-Irish were descendants of English nobility. The founding nobles had been given lands in

Ireland by English kings or queens as rewards for meritorious work, to become the landed gentry. The privilege, money and education of their descendants led them to become respected business leaders and professionals. Their strong sense of *noblesse oblige* led them, Peter said, "to became more Irish than the Irish," meaning they strongly supported many Irish causes. During Ireland's fight for independence from England in the early 1900s, their leadership effort earned them high marks and popularity. I felt immediately comfortable with these Anglo-Irish doctors, many educated in England, who followed medical standards like mine. Trinity College Dublin University, established by Queen Elizabeth I, was a bastion of Anglicans. Peter and I worked in the seven small Anglo-Irish affiliated hospitals where these doctors taught and practiced.

The dearth of laboratory tests required accurate diagnoses to be based on careful history and physical examination. Basic medicines and treatment procedures however, were available. One could generally practice good medicine this way, but I feared patients with complicated or rare diseases suffered. Infections, especially lung infections, were prevalent among the poor and unwashed public patients. Tuberculosis was so common it was the first illness one considered in any young person with chest symptoms and fever. Luckily, by this time we had antibiotics to treat them.

It also took me some time to get used to Irish patient attitudes. For instance, while an American patient wanted to know all the options from which he or she could choose, the Irish patient usually said, "You decide for me, Doctor." This compliance made it easier to do what I thought best, but burdened me with heavier responsibility.

Lack of resources often motivated improvisation. I purchased a special type of microscope and taught the laboratory technician how to identify crystals in joint fluid. We diagnosed and treated gout when we found uric acid crystals in several patients initially thought to have infected joints. With these limitations, Irish medicine was surprisingly good. Their national health system let patients pay according to their income, thereby providing medical care for everyone. If I had to find fault, I would say that while American doctors often erred by giving too many tests and treatments, the Irish doctors often erred by giving too few, and so lost patients who might have been saved.

Although Peter was very busy, we still enjoyed some relaxed time together. He never had time to sail in the Irish Sea, but we took walks along the Howth peninsula "cliff walk," and sat on rocks to watch the waves of the sea below. Farther south of Dublin, the Wicklow Mountains were another favorite place, and weekends often found us driving among the peat bogs that covered those mountains. Once we took a trip to county Clare on the west coast, where I fell in love with the Burren, an area of smooth sandstone rocks at the edge of the Atlantic Ocean. A spectacular variety of wild flowers grew in the moist cracks between the rocks. Botanists prized the pure blue gentians. To me, the beauty of Ireland lay in its natural loveliness in flowers, rocks, hills, skies and seas.

I was also fascinated by the lilting picturesque speech of the Irish. The engaging turn of phrase came naturally to them. In the pubs and at parties "the talk" went long into the night. Wonderful stories abounded, although one could never quite separate truth from fantasy. I had heard that the Irish could argue for hours about whether an angel could stand on the head of a pin, while maintaining interest and laughter. Peter used to say, "The Irish often substitute words for action." Not surprisingly all four Irish Nobel Prize laureates, W.B. Yeats, George Bernard Shaw, Samuel Beckett and Seamus Heaney, were for Literature. I was intrigued to discover several famous

Irish writers were Anglo-Irish—Jonathan Swift, George Bernard Shaw, James Joyce and Samuel Beckett. It appears this small group excelled in writing as well as in business and the professions. I recall receiving a phone call shortly after Peter's cousin Sam won the 1969 Nobel Prize. The unknown caller asked, "And are you related to Samuel Beckett, mum? You are? Why, all Ireland is basking in his reflected glory."

We had many acquaintances—medical colleagues, university teachers, and later after Peter became Dean of the Medical School, politicians and businessmen. But it was the few close friends who joined our dinners and trips in laughter and sorrow that immeasurably brightened our lives.

These are the sweet memories I have of Ireland.

Unwelcome outside world affairs intruded on our lives. Soon after our arrival, civil war erupted in Northern Ireland between the Protestant population who adhered to England, and the Catholic population who adhered to the southern Republic of Ireland. Most deaths took place in the north, but a few car bombs also went off down south where we lived. Later, during the worldwide oil shortage, Ireland's lack of natural sources of energy forced severe restrictions. We had to cut back on heating, and during gasoline rationing Peter started to bicycle to work. He said he didn't mind the commute, but missed our drives to his beloved Wicklow Mountains.

The deanship increased Peter's workload. He left for work at seven in the morning and often returned very tired about ten in the evening. After a brief supper he went straight to bed. Working from the dean's office during the day, he carried a portable dictaphone going from place to place with his assistant by his side. Because of daytime activities, the doctors and professors had to meet in the evenings to discuss administrative matters with Peter.

Based on his Mayo Clinic experience, Peter had the vision of merging and modernizing the hospitals and establishing a large outpatient clinic. This would require major alterations in the seven established hundred-year-old hospitals. Changing entrenched power and personnel is difficult in any country, but in Ireland the resistance to this change was especially fierce. Had the doctors not liked Peter so much, and realized it was to their benefit in the long run, they would never have gone along with his ambitious plans.

Sometimes Peter came home very frustrated. "I'm bound and determined to drag them kicking and screaming into the 20th century," he said. "When resistance becomes too intense, my ace in the hole is to say, 'Alright, have it your way. I'll go back to America.'" This, he chuckled, generally brought them around.

Because I saw him so little, I began leaving notes on his desk. I worried at this stepped-up pace, but he said he was fine. When he had a brief fainting spell soon after arriving in Ireland, I had urged him to check it out in America when he returned for psychiatric meetings. Two years earlier, he had been found well at the Mayo Clinic, so I said nothing. I was proud of all he was accomplishing and wanted to offer support in every way.

Then one early morning about five, I awoke to find him sitting up in bed in the dark. Turning the light on, I saw his right hand on the middle of his chest. He said, "I think I have indigestion from something I ate last night. I'll go downstairs and get some milk."

Quickly I said, "No, let me get it." I brought him the milk.

He drank it slowly and said, "That feels better. Thanks," as he lay back in bed. As I turned off the light, I thought, maybe he is getting an ulcer. I better get him to a doctor for a thorough exam.

A few minutes later, he suddenly said, "Hold my hand." Puzzled, I firmly gripped his hand. Then, feeling something was terribly wrong, I sat up and turned the light on again. His eyes were open, but he did not respond. His heart rate was grossly irregular and his pulse weak. Suddenly his heart stopped. I immediately started cardio-pulmonary resuscitation (CPR). No response. Again and again. No response. Only an electrical defibrillator could restart his heart. I dashed downstairs to the phone. Dublin had no 911, so I called a medical colleague to rush a cardiac ambulance with a defibrillator, then ran back upstairs to continue CPR. Still no response. His face became ashen; his skin grew cold. Dear God, no, I thought. Sometime later, our friend arrived with the ambulance. It was too late. The faithful heart that beat for fifty-one years finally stopped. My beloved Peter was gone forever.

My world collapsed. The sunlight went out of my life. I was empty and lost. Colleagues and friends overflowed the funeral service at the local Church of Ireland. Flanked by mountains of flowers, we laid his coffin in a hole in the ground on that bleak, cold, gray February day. I could not bear to leave him there, until someone dragged me home. My neighbors were there serving hot soup and sandwiches, while another friend brought whiskey. Slowly the conversation noise became cheerful as they laughed at stories about Peter. I vaguely felt Peter would have approved this Irish custom for he abhorred dreariness. When the Professor of Medicine, milling in the crowd, offered to interview me for a paying job, I became alert enough to book an appointment for the next week. Life had to go on, I told myself. There was no time to wallow in feelings.

I called my friend Ruth, the attorney in Michigan, to notify our various friends in America of Peter's death. Her immediate reply was, "Would you like me to come over? I could help you settle the estate."

"Would you?"

"Yes, of course," she said. "Both Irish and U.S. estate taxes could be troublesome."

"Oh, Ruth," I said, "It would be wonderful to have you here." This brought the first glimmer of hope in my grief and confusion.

"I will be in Dublin tomorrow afternoon. Don't bother to meet me. I shall rent a car at the airport and be at your doorstep late afternoon." And she was.

She drove me around Dublin in that rented car, step-by-step maneuvering me through the maze of gathering Peter's pension, and transferring property ownership and accounts. She also consulted with my Dublin lawyer. After she returned to Michigan she conferred with me weekly by phone or letter until the estate was settled on both sides of the Atlantic. Her prompt support gave me the strength and knowledge to put my affairs in order and to save the estate from unfair taxation. I owe her a debt I can never repay.

I initially planned to stay in Ireland to help continue some of Peter's work, but during the next two years, a succession of calamities finally crushed my hopes to do this. One evening about five-thirty I fell asleep while driving home from work. My car swerved, sideswiped another car, then tipped over on its side. Bystanders righted my car and pulled me out. Neither the woman and her son in the other car, nor I were hurt, but the side of her car was crushed in. I did not mind the brief court hearing and small fine, but the judge refused to let me drive again until a neurologic exam excluded epilepsy as a possible cause for the accident. After an anxious three months using inconvenient public transport, I was finally allowed to drive again.

Six months after Peter's death I developed iritis, an immune inflammation of the eye of unknown cause. Cortisone drops controlled it, but it was a nuisance and I feared losing my vision.

Another day I discovered a breast lump, which to my relief, turned out to be benign on surgical biopsy. About then, I accidentally singed my eyebrows and front hair when a gas oven I was lighting exploded in my face. Another time, I inadvertently left the second floor bathroom faucet dripping. Two hours later when I returned, I opened the front door to find the first floor covered with an inch of water. The upstairs bathroom had flooded, and the water had dripped down through the ceiling to the floor below. What a mess to clean up. I felt jinxed.

The first Christmas after my husband's death, I drove with my fourteen-year-old son to Christmas dinner at St. Patrick Hospital, and parked in the hospital parking lot. After a pleasant dinner celebration, we came out to find my car gone—stolen.

The *garda* (policeman) said, "If you don't get the car back in twenty-four hours, it's gone for good. It'll be taken over the border to become a car bomb."

At two in the morning the phone rang. It was the garda.

"We found your car, mum. Its been stripped but you can still drive it. You'll have to remove it, or by morning every bit of it will be stolen, tires and all." He gave me an address in the worst part of Dublin.

I pleaded, "Can't you move it to the police station, so I can pick it up in the morning?"

"No, mum, you'll have to do what you can." He hung up.

In desperation I phoned Automobile Association of Ireland. A cheerful male voice answered. When I explained my predicament, he said, "Sure now, I can tow the car back for you. It'll take me an hour or two." At three-thirty that morning, my towed car appeared at our driveway, minus radio, minus contents of trunk and glove compartment, with an empty gas tank and a broken window. When that AA man came into my living room to have me sign papers, he saw my piano, and to my utter astonishment, insisted on playing some songs he had composed. He turned out to be a musician earning money by working at the AA, so at three-thirty a.m. I was listening to him play bright, catchy tunes! From feeling battered and bruised I began smiling again. Next day, my local garage promptly repaired the car damage. Looking back, it was typical of so many memories of Ireland—a mixture of laughter and tears.

The continued oil crisis limited driving and often meant living in the dark and cold, a grimness lasting several months. During the next two years, I continued teaching and practicing medicine as before, but now had the additional salaried post of post-graduate director of the Dublin Federated Hospitals. In this post I organized a matching program for medical school graduates to apply to these seven hospitals for further training, similar to the American system. It worked well to the benefit of both graduates and hospitals.

One afternoon, I received a phone call from the matron of my son's boarding school.

"Please go to the Adelaide Hospital to sign permission for minor surgery on Paul's finger. Don't worry, he's all right. A glass sliver is embedded in his finger from a broken chemistry class beaker. We couldn't remove it in the dispensary, so we sent him to the hospital." I promptly called Ann, my sister-in-law, to cancel our dinner engagement. She insisted on driving me to the hospital. Passing through downtown Dublin on the way, we were stopped in a street jammed with cars. A garda with a bull horn waved us back.

"Go back! Go back! A bomb is about to go off!"

I shouted to Ann, "Let's leave the car and run."

Without a word, she made a U-turn onto the sidewalk, then drove along an alley to eventually reach the Adelaide. Paul was sitting up in bed with his bandaged hand in a sling, watching television beside three men who shared his room. We all watched the carnage of the car bomb explosion which we had just escaped. God surely watched over us that night!

All widows must feel doors closing around them as attitudes change. My status plummeted after Peter's death. The final blow was when my eye doctor referred to me as "Professor Beckett's widow." As an Asian, a woman and an American, I was definitely an outsider. In a land where local people fought fiercely for the few available jobs, there was no place for me. All these calamities seemed to be God telling me, "Go back to America where you can make a life of your own." I listened.

I had shared a wonderful twenty years with a remarkable man, and had spent seven of them in his native land. It was time to take my son back to America where we belonged.

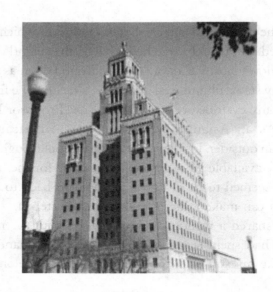

Mayo Clinic in Plummer Building, 1953

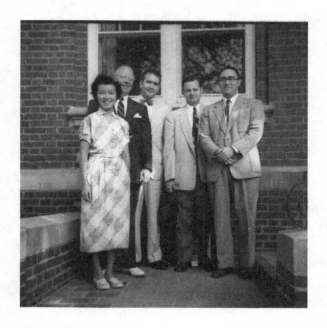

Dr. E. Rynearson and medical residents,
outside Worrall Hospital, Rochester,MN

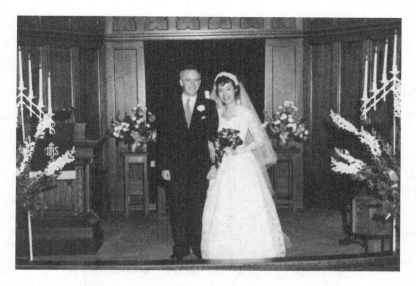

Wedding with Dr. Peter G.S. Beckett, Rochester, MN, 1954

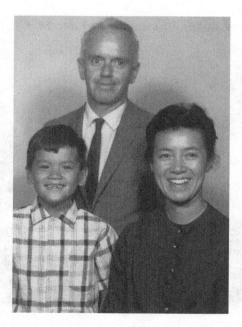

Beckett family, husband Peter and son Paul,
Detroit, MI. 1966.

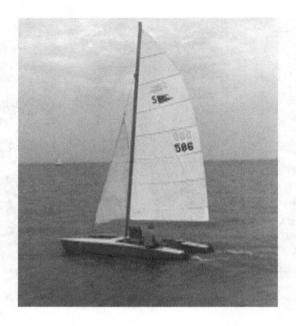

Husband Peter sailing in catamaran, Lake St. Clair, MI 1966.

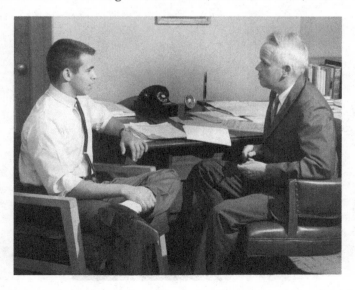

Husband Peter, Assistant Director of Lafayette Clinic,
with psychiatry resident, Detroit, MI

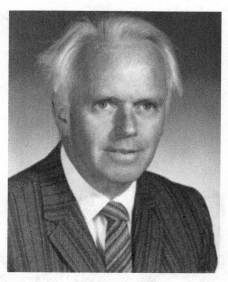

Husband Peter, Professor and first Chairman of Psychiatry
Dept., Trinity College Medical School, Dublin, Ireland.
In 1973 also Dean of Medical School

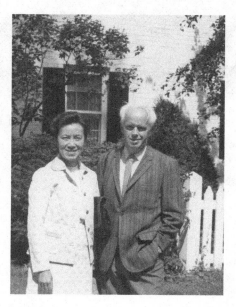

Husband Peter and author revisit Detroit, 1972.

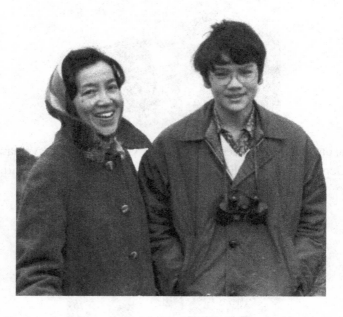

Son Paul and author visit with friends West Coast of Ireland, 1974

Chapter 12

ROCHESTER, MN:
THE MAYO TRADITION 1976-90

Impatient to resume my professional life in the U.S., I decided to attend a medical meeting at Mayo in Rochester, Minnesota. Along the way, I hoped to explore job opportunities in New York and Michigan where I had connections. In Michigan I stopped to visit my attorney friend, Ruth, who surprised me by asking, "Have you applied for a job at Mayo?"

"No, I'm just attending a medical meeting. I have little chance of getting a job there, considering how long I've been away."

"Well, why not apply? It can't hurt," she said.

She was right. I typed out an application and mailed it immediately.

A week later, I was warmly greeted at the Rochester airport by my old friends, Maurie and Shirley Barry, who took me to stay in their familiar home. In the evening after we were settled, Maurie, to my amazement, handing me a schedule the Mayo Clinic asked him to give me. It included interviews with various Mayo division chiefs, staff physicians, administrators and even the financial officer. After three days of interviews, I was offered the position of staff physician (called "consultant"), to work in either Rheumatology or Area Medicine divisions. Elated, I selected my field of Rheumatology. Dr. Howard Polley, chief of the Rheumatology division, granted me six months to wind up affairs in Ireland.

In June 1976 my son and I returned to America. This time, my friends, Jane Duncan and Shirley Barry, met us at the Rochester airport. Jane was now a Mayo staff pediatric psychiatrist. We had been medical school classmates, and later residents-in-training at Mayo at the same time. After introducing my son to her three sons, she filled me in on changes at the Mayo Clinic and in the city of Rochester. Shirley gave me a key to a furnished terrace apartment in southeast Rochester with a one-year rental lease.

A few days later I started work in the familiar Mayo system with a heart-warming welcome by my former mentors and peers. They made me feel I had come home. I had old friends here, happy memories and I was proud to be part of this splendid place again.

Unlike my status as a resident-in-training in the 1950s, I was now a staff physician with full responsibility for my patients, and represented the institution to the outside world. I reviewed again the basic principles that had so successfully guided all Mayo activities.

- The *patient* is the primary focus, and must receive the highest standard of medical care regardless of race, gender, creed or income.
- All the professionals, including the medical physicians, surgeons and laboratory scientists are to work in a coordinated *team* to provide total care for each patient.
- The institution should *continue in perpetuity* through its organizational infrastructure, educational and research programs.

- Necessary *financial* management must maintain the institution, but no patient should be asked to pay beyond his or her ability. There would be no financial benefit for staff or employee beyond reasonable annual compensation, and only enough return to the institution to safeguard its future.

I knew I could happily devote my life to an organization with such ideals.

How such an institution came into being is an astonishing story in itself. In 1863 Dr. William Worrall Mayo (the father) arrived in Rochester to be the examining surgeon of the Civil War draft board for southern Minnesota, and he stayed on after the war to practice medicine. He raised two sons, William James (born 1861) and Charles Horace (born 1865), who worked alongside him, and later attended first class medical schools. When a tornado ripped through Rochester in 1883, all three worked tirelessly to care for the injured. They persuaded the local teaching nuns of St. Frances to help as nurses. Later, the doctors worked together to establish the Mayo Clinic for outpatient care, and at the nuns' insistence, teamed together with them to establish St. Mary's Hospital to provide surgery and inpatient care. The two brothers' amazing surgical skill first brought medical fame to Rochester. But it was Dr. William J. Mayo's vision of this country's first private group practice that created this renowned medical center. His brother, Dr. Charles Mayo and the inventive internal medicine physician, Dr. Henry Plummer, also contributed in important ways. Although both Mayo brothers died in 1939, their spirit still permeates the institution— nearly every medical meeting is inspired by quotations from their writing and speaking.

My typical workday demonstrates how the daily tasks and responsibilities of a staff physician reflects the Mayo principles.

In 1976 about eight hundred full-time staff physicians and their residents-in-training, saw about a thousand patients a day. The graceful Italianate-style Plummer Building had been replaced by a modern twenty-story gray marble, cross-shaped Mayo Clinic Building, that occupied an entire square block. Its basic interior arrangement was the same as before—each floor had a central patient lobby, corridors of examining rooms, front desks, medical record area and secretarial rooms. Its clean, modern, straight-line décor included huge ten-by-thirty-four foot murals on each floor with titles like: Man and Recreation, Man and Plant Forms, Man and Sea, Earth and Sky. Although the enlargement sacrificed some of the family intimacy of the 1950s, the quality of patient care remained high.

Most patients took a week to "go through the Clinic." Each weekday morning I conducted three to four full general medical work-ups of new patients. I spent afternoons reviewing test results and outlining a course of treatment to each patient. Throughout the day, I inserted brief fifteen-minute "Priority Interviews" to triage walk-in patients without appointments.

All patients were welcome. An example was the story of a science colleague. He said, "Many years ago, as a young man in Minneapolis between jobs, I dropped by to see what this Mayo Clinic was all about before heading west. I asked for a physical exam. There were many reasons the Clinic could have refused—I had no physician referral, no job, no funds, not even a known illness. None of this seemed to matter while I received a full examination. To my consternation a neck tumor was found. The doctor carefully explained its implications. With my consent, an eminent surgeon promptly removed it the next day. I've had no trouble from it since. I simply wasn't prepared for the kindness, courtesy and good medical care I received. Only after recuperation did the business office work out a fair repayment schedule. You can guess what I think of Mayo even today."

For me the best part of the day was the friendly interaction with other consultants. We consulted on arthritic problems for colleagues in other specialties, and they helped us from their specialty knowledge. We learned from each other as we discussed cases, and provided the patient with our best combined opinions. This interaction also kept us on our toes, since our colleagues could certainly see how we cared for our patients. Since we were all on salary, we did not compete for patients, but worked together. It has been said, "A single Mayo physician may not stand out, but as a team they are unsurpassed."

My patient with a curious right arm pain illustrated this. I initially thought he had coronary disease heart pain, but he kept saying, "It hurts most when my arm hangs down by my side." This was not characteristic of heart pain. His shoulder and chest x-rays were normal, as was his electrocardiogram. A neurologist colleague found nerve damage in his arm but could not pinpoint its source. Then a cardiovascular colleague suggested a tomogram, a special x-ray image, to show an area above the right collar bone that is obscured in routine chest x-rays. He was right on target. The tomogram disclosed a small lung tumor exactly at the site that pressed on nerves traveling from the shoulder area down the arm causing the pain.

I also worked closely with surgical colleagues. The Clinic required a thorough medical examination before each surgery to minimize surgical risk and to free the surgeons from complex medical evaluations. After the patient passed my medical exam, I would introduce him or her to a surgeon. The surgeon would then decide whether to proceed with surgery, and if so, what type. Once surgery was elected, with the patient's consent, the procedure was usually scheduled for the next day and the patient whisked to the hospital.

Even patients directly referred to Mayo surgeons for specific surgery must have a brief preoperative medical clearance. I usually approved these cases after about a fifteen-minute evaluation of their lab tests and general physical condition, but occasionally I had to pursue more urgent medical problems. A rheumatoid arthritis patient was very displeased when I delayed her hip surgery to evaluate her anemia. A right colon cancer causing the anemia was found, and it had to be removed before her hip could be repaired.

In the area of teaching, I supervised residents' care of patients throughout the day. It was stimulating to discuss problems with these bright young minds. Most of us also enjoyed teaching medical students, so several times a year, I taught them general physical diagnosis, or examination of the joints. In the area of clinical research, I was encouraged to specialize on one disease entity, to develop a special niche of expertise. I chose scleroderma[17]. My drug studies on these patients generated several research papers.

Since my resident days, Rheumatology had changed to include a large group of very sick patients with connective tissue diseases from obscure immune mechanisms. They have been most challenging to treat; lupus and scleroderma are among such diseases.

A pleasant chore was conducting "Executive Exams" of business executives. These healthy adults wanted speedy check-

---

[17] Scleroderma: a connective tissue disease where patients develop generalized skin thickening, deficient blood supply to the fingers, and often later, lung fibrosis and kidney failure.

ups. I previewed their completed questionnaires and scheduled specific laboratory tests and consultations to promptly start on their arrival. The following day, I carried out a physical exam and reviewed their laboratory results. I rarely found medical problems needing further assessment. These men and women were extremely bright and pleasant to deal with, and frequently came and left as a group in a corporate jet.

In addition to weekly morning, noon or evening medical meetings to attend, we were asked to join various committees to help run the Clinic. I chose our division education committee that met monthly to monitor and discuss our teaching duties for residents and medical students. The more important institutional Standing Committees monitored specific endeavors for the entire Clinic, but I did not belong to any of them. For example, in proposing my scleroderma study project, I had to first persuade our division research committee of its merits. Then the Institutional Review Board (a powerful standing committee) checked on the project's ethical, safety, legal and financial aspects, before they gave me approval to proceed.

We were expected to maintain careful records for each patient we saw, and to send a detailed report of tests, treatments and suggestions to their referring physicians. On free evenings and weekends, I dictated these summary letters, worked on my research project and read specialty medical journals.

Two breaks in this Clinic routine were hospital service and outside medical meetings. When I started, our division had three hospital units, two at St. Mary's Hospital, one at Methodist Hospital. During the year, we were scheduled to rotate, a month at a time, to full-time hospital service on any one of the hospital units. Hospital service emphasized bedside supervising and teaching of residents, as we together cared for very sick bed patients. The Clinic encouraged attendance at out-of-state medical meetings, to present papers and to learn. This "cross-fertilization" prevented inbreeding. I loved meeting other physicians, listening to new medical ideas and visiting new places. In fact, I often extended my stay one or two days to roam in a new city. In this way, I have visited most major U.S. cities, as well as many Mediterranean and Scandinavian cities.

The Mayo way and culture is quite distinctive. The Mayo brothers broke new ground when they created a private group practice and put all physicians on salaries. Although the salaries are not as high as in individual private practice, they are fair and the pensions and perks generous. I particularly appreciate the competent administrative staff who run the onerous business side of the institution, freeing me to concentrate wholly on patient care and professional activities.

The Clinic's central control is strong yet flexible, maintaining standards but allowing change. All consultants are considered equal partners, and given the opportunity to participate, grow and innovate according to our ability and interests. This is not to say there are no disagreements, jealousies or mistakes, but they are resolved, mostly amicably, without damage to the institution. The constant encouragement to do more and better brings out the best in us.

I have been asked if I ever felt discrimination at work, probably referring to gender discrimination, although racial or ethnic discrimination may also have been implied. As a woman physician of Chinese birth, who worked at the Mayo Clinic for seventeen years, I can truthfully answer, "Never." Colleagues and nonprofessional staff have always treated me with the complete equality and courtesy all Mayo physicians receive. Frankly, I rarely think of myself as Chinese or a woman, but simply as a professional striving to be a good physician. Perhaps a big help has been avoiding a victim role and spending my life in academic and professional circles where diversity prevails.

The more important issue was the patient's attitude toward me. Sometimes a patient looked startled when I walked in the door and introduced myself, "I am your physician, Dr. Beckett." They did not expect either a woman or an Asian. I would immediately allay their concerns by saying if they were uncomfortable with me for any reason, I would be glad to call another physician. At this, they seemed reassured, and by the time they recited their symptoms their initial concern had evaporated. Conversely, women patients sometimes requested me, preferring a woman physician.

However, I tried to forestall trouble. Occasionally when a male patient had a difficult urology problem, or had an ethnic background which might make him uncomfortable with a woman physician, I would have him switched to a male colleague. One time I was not quick enough, when in walked a high official from a Middle East nation. His interpreter and he brushed aside my suggestion of another physician as he poured out his medical troubles. He had ankylosing spondylitis, an arthritic condition of the spine that causes pain and stiffness. Although there is no cure for the condition, a number of symptomatic treatments are helpful. After undergoing his treatment regimen, I had a pleased and grateful patient.

Another time, as I entered the room, a pale, heavy-set man in his late sixties, sitting on the patient couch, brusquely announced, "I sue doctors!" He was a lawyer from the south with both severe coronary disease and extreme hypothyroidism (subnormal thyroid function). Bringing his thyroid status up to normal with thyroid pills aggravated his coronary angina pain, so his treatment required a delicate balance between the two conditions. Fortunately I earned his trust enough to help him maintain this balance for several years. One day I was saddened to received a letter from his sister notifying me of his death, but she wanted to emphasize how much he appreciated my care.

Looking back on my time as staff consultant at the Clinic, I recall intense personal feelings and thoughts. When I began as a Mayo consultant in 1976, I felt inadequate to be at the cutting edge of medicine in this great institution after my uneven practice in Detroit and Dublin. I vowed to devote my total energy to becoming a top-notch Mayo physician in gratitude for their confidence in me. Nevertheless, I was not prepared for the demanding patient needs that taxed my mental, emotional and physical stamina. Sometimes the whole world seemed sick. Neither had I expected the agonizing self-doubt over difficult decisions for a patient, the devastating self-torment over mistakes, nor the deep sorrow when one of my patients died. On the other hand, there were also times of tremendous satisfaction when a patient recovered or improved.

In spite of the stresses, I thoroughly enjoyed the stimulating work, the comradeship with colleagues and dealing with all kinds of patients. I found solving both simple and complex diagnostic cases fascinating. A list of my colleagues, from all over the U.S. as well as overseas, reads like a roll call in the United Nations. I have been happy to call many of these talented people my friends. Patients too were a diverse group. Most were solid farming people of Scandinavian origin from the surrounding five-state Midwest area. Many also came from South America and Canada, fewer from Europe and a trickle from Asia and the Middle East. Dealing with people of such varied backgrounds was ever interesting and challenging.

With time, I gained confidence in my own abilities. But above all, I was tremendously proud of being part of the Mayo Clinic. This same feeling was shared from consultants to janitors, and was reflected in our legendary expertise and kindness toward patients. Extremely low personnel turnover rate gives the Clinic a loyal work force, providing a strong institution with a happy working atmosphere.

Over the years I have seen many changes at the Clinic. Increasing numbers of bright young women are earning staff positions. The Mayo medical school has contributed new residents and later staff physicians to the Clinic. Increasing specialization has occurred in both medicine and surgery.

In internal medicine, we now have available a vast array of antibiotics and hormones, the recognition of the puzzling and challenging immune phenomena, multiple effective drugs for numerous medical conditions, and much more. In the laboratory field there is a host of sophisticated biochemical tests and new imaging techniques to expedite more accurate diagnoses. In surgery, new and better surgical techniques are saving more lives, and lengthening others. The rise in short-stay surgery, such as for cataracts and gallstones, has reduced patient discomfort and costs. The success of joint replacement has given people increased mobility. Diseased kidneys, heart and other organs are increasingly transplanted.

Medical records have followed the move into the electronic age. As more patients push to come, buildings are enlarged and new ones completed. The Clinic now has two sister clinics, one in Florida, the other in Arizona, and we have merged with a dozen small medical practices in adjacent towns and states. As we enter the exciting era of the genome, medicine will change in ways we cannot yet imagine. Nevertheless, to quote a colleague, "Our task is still basically the same, to sit across from the patient, one-on-one, listen to him and help whenever we can."

Throughout all the changes in a hundred-year history, the ideals of the Mayo brothers have been the solid foundation of the Clinic's practice. Chiseled into the pink and white marble wall at the entry lobby of the Siebens Building (next to the Plummer Building) are their words:

> *There are two objects of medical education: to heal the sick and to advance the science.*
>
> Charles H. Mayo

> *The glory of medicine is that it is constantly moving forward, that there is always more to learn.*
>
> William J. Mayo

Wonderful as my Mayo years have been, more exciting things were still to happen.

Chapter 13

RETIREMENT:

EXPLORATION, PHYSICAL PATHS 1990-

2000

After forty years practicing medicine, retirement brought both happy anticipation and trepidation. Realizing it would take time to reorient myself to a completely different life, I took nearly two years to plan this change—first when to retire, then what to do in retirement.

Although sixty-five was the standard retirement age at the Clinic, under certain circumstances we could postpone it a while, although part-time work was not then an option. I repeatedly asked myself three questions:

- Can I feel self-worth if I am no longer practicing medicine?
- Can I find other meaningful activities to devote my life to?
- Will I have adequate funds for my retirement years?

When I felt I could answer "Yes" to all three, I retired.

On July 24, 1990 colleagues in the Rheumatology Division gave me a splendid retirement party at the imposing Mayo

Foundation House. After saying nice things about me, they presented me with a heavy, solid silver engraved dinner tray. I recall thanking them for their help and inspiration in the years we worked together. Then I added, "In my Christian belief, I have always wondered what was more important—'Being' or 'Doing,' and I've concluded both are. Well, after all these years of 'Doing' I am now going to concentrate on 'Being.' Having learned so much about the human body, I now want to learn about human emotions and the human spirit, and how they apply to me. I would like to create and enjoying beauty, as in the arts and in my efforts in cooking." I ended with, "Don't be surprised to be invited for dinner and a good chat."

Next came the formal retirement ceremonies at the November Annual Mayo Staff Dinner at the Civic Center, when new staff were announced and retiring staff honored. I sat on the platform among thirty new emeriti colleagues. When our names were intoned, we each rose to hear a summary of our Mayo work and to be presented with an elaborately hand-inscribed leather folder. My son attended wearing a new suit, and gave me a big hug. Later I received a gold Longine wrist watch that I prize for the memories it evokes.

For six wonderful months, I relished the freedom from appointments, getting up late, reading the *Wall Street Journal* at breakfast, and visiting with friends and relatives. Except for paying a few bills, I refused to do anything serious.

But after this time of idleness, I grew bored. The Clinic had generosity provided an Emeritus Office—a suite of rooms in the Plummer Building—to help transition from total immersion in medicine. Three secretaries handled our letters and mail. We were assigned shared offices (with file drawers), and given the run of a lounge room (with newspapers and snacks), a computer room, a meeting room and dictation cubicles. We could and did, continue attending the various meetings of our interest held all over the Clinic. But soon this too was not enough. There was no challenge in being just a spectator.

To start "Being" I decided to explore what was possible, what I liked and what would be meaningful to me. I was in good health and my son was away at university, so I was free to try many avenues. I planned first to concentrate on maintaining my physical well-being, then my mental and financial well-being. Afterward, I needed to resolve several emotional issues, and finally, I would focus on my spiritual quest. Since I was no longer working, I wanted to do something different and fun, so I could continue feeling I had something to offer others. These distinct realms of activities became intertwined in practice.

Having been blessed with good health, I had never thought much about it during my working years. Now recognizing my advancing age, I decided to improve some of my habits, starting with diet and exercise.

How could I make my diet healthier without gaining weight? Working full-time and living alone, I had paid scant attention to meals—soups and sandwiches were the norm. By chance, a colleague, Dr. Joe Sharp, had just finished a two-week workshop in California on the Pritikin Method for a healthy life. An enthusiastic convert, he loaned me the Pritikin recipe book, authored by a French chef, to produce delicious dishes low in cholesterol, fat and salt. Although I had sent many patients to our dietitians for instructions to reduce cholesterol levels, I had never attempted such diets myself. Since I loved to cook, I thought it would be challenging to try new ways of buying, cooking and eating. Besides, my new friend offered to try out the new dishes.

I quickly discovered I had to decrease or omit less healthy foods, such as butter, cream, eggs and salty or fatty meats. But

I could replace them with skim milk, low fat cheese, yogurt, egg substitute or soy milk. I should limit beef and pork to the leanest cuts, and increase intake of chicken and turkey. Fish dishes were encouraged, and I learned to love broiled salmon. The best cooking oils were canola or olive oil. To avoid frying foods, I could bake, broil, stir-fry or steam. Spices and herbs could be added to give taste to low salt dishes.

Also recommended were more vegetables, fruits and starches. Many forms of beans entered my dishes, including kidney beans in chili, mashed refried beans and different types of canned beans. I grew especially fond of garbanzo beans and lentil soups. Fresh peas, pea pods and stir-fried string beans were very tasty, and I doubled quantities of leafy and root vegetables at every meal.

Fruits became a delightful replacement for richer desserts and snacks. Available were bananas, apples and grapes throughout the year, and strawberries, blueberries, peaches, apricots, pears and melons in season. Fresh pineapple and pink Florida grapefruit were special treats. For starches, I cooked mixtures of white and healthy brown rice, potatoes in every form, varieties of pasta, and I bought the best freshly baked whole-grain bread from local bakeries—oat bran, whole wheat, pumpernickel or rye. Later, as diet recommendations changed, I cut down on starches and added more meat and vegetables, limiting my daily total calories to about 1500 (for my five-feet-one and one-hundred-and-ten pounds). Making these changes took time and effort, but my healthier dishes were soon as delicious as previous ones.

Just as a test, I demonstrated these ideas at a local organic food store. Using an electric frying pan I cooked Pineapple Chicken Stir-fry and Ratatouille Eggplant Medley. I also made half-and-half white/brown rice mixture in an electric rice-cooker. Some of the attending crowd returned to tell me they really liked the taste of the food. Although I had a ready taster in Joe, I enlarged the taster group by giving parties at home with gratifying success. I plan to continue such enjoyable parties.

The other side of physical health involves exercise. How was a person who had never exercised beyond daily housework, gardening and snow shoveling supposed to start? I heard of a Mayo MD, PhD candidate who was an excellent black belt teacher of Tae Kwon-do, a Korean form of martial arts. He taught both adult and children classes, so I went to watch a children class for beginners. A dozen eight-to-ten year old boys and girls stood at attention on a large polished wooden floor. They wore white cotton kimono-like clothes tied with yellow belts (lowest order). Facing them stood their teacher, Tom, five-feet-ten, short haircut, glasses and an infectious smile, who was similarly dressed but with a black belt (highest order). At his signal, the students formally bowed to him and he returned their bow; then they chanted in unison, "We will show *obedienc*e to our teacher, *help* for fellow students and *respect* for the class of Tae Kwon-do"—a remarkable scene in Middle America. As he barked orders, he demonstrated sequential fluid movements of disciplined force. Striving to imitate him, the children seemed to welcome his strict discipline as they proudly went through their movements.

I was so impressed I signed up for an eight-week adult beginner class. Unlike judo, Tae Kwon-do is not a strenuous, aggressive exercise, but a set of slower, gentler, disciplined movements. Following these movements left me a little breathless, but not aching or tired. At first, I didn't think I could ever master all the sequential moves. Nevertheless, I practiced them at every chance, at home, in a classmate's apartment and after class with the teacher assistants. Suddenly one day I found

I had learned them all. Then came the dramatic high point of the eight-week class—each member of the class was individually tested by three judges in front of the whole class. I carefully carried out each required movement. To my delight, I passed to earn an orange belt. Next came the green belt, then the blue, the brown and the red belts—each requiring more advanced movements. The red belt (just before the black, the highest order) required breaking boards with one's feet. Afraid that my foot bones might break in the process, I regretfully dropped out of further classes. But I had learned physical discipline, the importance of regular practice, the thrill of accomplishing complex body movements and the wonderful sensation of lightness and health after exercising.

I then experimented with other forms of exercises. Six months of ballet convinced me it was not for me. By great good fortune, I next tried a Stretch class at a local athletic club, and knew immediately it was what I had been looking for—part exercise, part fluid movement, neither following a progressive schedule nor performance for an audience. It was non-aggressive and non-aerobic (does not increase heart rate), physical yet had a spiritual quality. Best of all, it promoted flexibility, balance and grace. The instructor, Jane, a tall, attractive, agile brunette, showed us how graceful we could become as we learned a series of stretching movements to the rhythm of soft, slow music. I learned the routines as a student, taught them as a teacher assistant, and finally became a full-fledged teacher creating my own routines.

When Mayo opened their Healthy Living Center, I went there to teach. I added to my repertoire by studying Yoga with an experienced Korean teacher and Tai-chi under two Chinese instructors. Tai-chi is a defensive Chinese martial art, resembling a slow-motion dance. Buddhist Yoga consists of holding certain poses for specified periods. These poses range from simple to complex, some twisting the individual like a corkscrew. Eventually I combined these disciplines into an hour-long class—the first half Tai-chi and the last half Yoga and Stretch. This worked the students from head to toe, from easy to difficult poses. My experience as a rheumatologist helped me design poses to improve flexibility while avoiding injury. I played slow background music to encourage students to move slowly. I urged even the least athletic students to attend regularly, so they could gain better posture and move more easily. Better yet, these types of exercises could be continued for the rest of their lives.

The class response was a joy. An excited, overweight young woman approached me after class. "I didn't think I could do these exercises, but I can follow you. It feels great." A gray-haired, slightly stooped woman stopped me one morning to say, "My husband kept telling me to stand up straight, but I never listened. Now after being in your class, he tells me I am straighter, and even a little taller." An Indian gentleman told me he had learned Yoga as a youth, but neglected it when he became busy at work. In my class he relearned many poses and was feeling more fit. These have been my rewards. I continue to teach because it keeps me in good shape and I enjoy it. Surprisingly, I found planning and executing new routines quite easy and pleasant. As an Asian, I naturally felt kinship with these Eastern forms of exercise. But the best news is many unfit and older persons have found an exercise class they can master and like. I am anxious to keep abreast of emerging alternative types of exercise that could benefit this group.

I rediscovered the gardening I had neglected during my working years. It has been a joy to dig the brown earth in the fresh outdoors under sunny skies, with only the sound of birds singing and bees buzzing around me. As my Irish mother-in-law used to say, "Gardening is like working next to God." It has been most satisfying to plant, care for and watch plants grow. I asked a local gardening center to landscape my home by planting evergreens and outlining flower planting areas around my house, leaving a birch tree and two crab apples trees at strategic spots. I inserted annuals, such as marigolds, petunias, violets and begonias between perennials, such as irises, daylilies, roses and clematis. This provided a variety of colors, with something coming into bloom each month of the growing season. A gardening friend with a yen for phlox and asters, persuaded me to plant her cuttings. Their pinks, purples and whites contrasted nicely with the yellow chrysanthemums in the fall. I loved looking out the kitchen window to see this panorama of bright colors. Later, copying my next-door neighbor's large vegetable garden, I added tomatoes, green peppers and zucchini plants in a garden corner. Their bountiful yields with almost no care helped me eat well those summers. The good exercise in gardening was an added bonus.

Improving these physical aspects in my life has helped me sleep better, maintain a normal weight and feel better than ever before.

Chapter 14

RETIREMENT:

MENTAL PATHS 1990-2000

Having satisfied my goals for health, I now intended to explore ways to continue my mental well-being. I had seen so many older people give up, feeling they were no longer important, and lose interest in their surroundings and current events. Worse, some even began to lose memory and judgement. As a firm believer of the dictum, "If you don't use it, you lose it," I was determined to ward off as many of these changes as possible by engaging in thought-provoking activities.

Living close to the Rochester University Center made college the natural starting place. What courses should I take? To widen my knowledge of the creative arts, I chose a Music Appreciation class. Arriving on campus in my business suit and brief case, I felt conspicuously out of place, so I switched to shirt, slacks and backpack to mingle with the eighteen-year olds. The years seemed to slip away.

The music teacher was a round-faced, earnest young man with glasses and straight brown ear-length hair. He asked us to memorize dates of specific musical periods, such as Baroque 1600-1750, Classical 1750-1800, Romantic 1800-1910 and so on up to the present. Different world events influenced the music of each period. While playing music from various periods, he described the specific musical changes as well as the newly introduced musical instruments. He said, "You may not like each type of music, but I want you to listen carefully to each piece and try to understand what the composers of the time wanted to say." Using loan tapes at home to study each era by its music, I was surprised to find the exercise both difficult and interesting. Near the end of term, we were asked to attend an evening concert of the Rochester Symphony Orchestra, and write a critique on both the musical quality and audience reaction. I had attended many such concerts before, but never had I probed them in such depths nor felt such an enriching experience.

I also found a way to experience modern rock music. I persuaded a male friend to accompany me to a local bar—a place I had previously shunned. In a dimly lit room, the three electric guitar players and a drummer produced deafening sounds with a strong beat, while dancers on the crowded floor accompanied the beat with strenuous, uninhibited movements. It reminded me of a strange, primitive tribal scene. When I finished the term, I felt I had really learned to listen and appreciate different types of music.

This led to the purchase of an electronic piano to restart the piano lessons that had lapsed since my teenage days. My patient piano teacher encouraged me to keep practicing until I achieved some proficiency. Although a beginner, I prefer pieces by Bach with its subtle intertwining contrapuntal lines. I have begun pausing during the day to play the piano. This helps me appreciate periods of beauty in the midst of a busy day. How nice I can plan to continue in this way.

Next, came a class in Creative Writing. My mother, an English teacher, started my fascination with the English language when I was a young girl in China. After arriving in America, learning to speak and write good English became a necessity and a pleasure. My first college English paper was "Origins of the English Language," where I learned its unusual expressiveness flowed from its many foreign sources—Greek, Latin, French and German. My medical years had taught me to write in the third person, passive voice, and in medical jargon. Now to reach a wide lay audience, this was no longer appropriate. I embarked on learning a new way of writing—in non-fiction narrative genre. Journalist-historian Barbara Tuchman became my model. I felt any author who could rivet me to a war book like *The Guns of August* was worthy to emulate.

I eventually took four writing classes and one journalism class. In a writing class, the teacher asked us to submit essays on the same subject written in the first, second and third persons, then in present and past tenses, and finally in short pithy words and in long elegant words. The differences were quite astounding. Other teachers taught us to adhere to an overall theme, omit needless words, be specific and concrete, avoid cliches, "show, don't tell," use dialogue to enliven narrative and so on. We studied samples writings of famous authors and also read books on how to write. Among the latter, my favorites were by William Zinsser, William Strunk and E.B White, Jerome Stern, Brenda Ueland and Gary Provost. I wrote essay after essay, gradually improving. In the process, I learned to use the computer, which became a familiar and essential writing tool.

In journalism class I studied the art of interview and its write-up. I had to read newspapers, such as *New York Times, Wall Street Journal, Rochester Post-Bulletin,* and news magazines, such as *Time, U.S. News & World Report.* I learned to discern bias and accuracy, as well as to note how events and opinions could be presented. I even interviewed a city official and wrote it up.

Slowly I developed my own writing style. I then enrolled in a year-long correspondence writing course that taught me to write and submit articles for magazine publication. While improving my writing style, it also taught me how difficult it is to get published. But once I started writing I could not stop. The sheer joy of putting delicious words and provocative thoughts on paper has kept me closely on this path.

By chance I was introduced to "We Care," a self-help support group for widows, divorced and single people. Unexpectedly, I found their approach gave real help to those who participated. But delving into people's emotional life without formal training troubled me, so I enrolled in a Psychology class on human development. The many new findings about the human mind and emotions from birth to death caught my attention. This led to my taking classes at St. Mary's University, Rochester branch toward a Masters degree in Human Development with an emphasis on psychology and creative writing. Eighteen months of concentrated work, including classes in neuro-anatomy, statistics and conducting a controlled study of support groups for rheumatoid patients resulted in a Master of Arts degree.

This work helped me appreciate how strongly emotions influence our health. I became convinced a positive attitude was essential for patients to cope with daily discomforts, especially those with chronic diseases. Most acute illnesses can be cured by appropriate medicines or surgery, so the majority of the long-term patients doctors see today are those with chronic illnesses. They carry on with only treatment of their symptoms. I believe a Complementary Alternative Medicine program to augment their standard medical treatment will greatly improve their quality of life. This would include self-help support groups, regular mild exercise such as Tai-chi, a good healthy diet, information on herbs, therapeutic massage and trials of acupuncture and other non-invasive pain relieving procedures. I have urged the Mayo Clinic to try such a program, which other medical centers have already begun. Now a new Mayo website has started the interactive dialogue part—support groups, diets and information on herbs. In the Clinic, cancer support groups have sprung up, and physician consultations on herbs and diets are available. Moreover, patients can now be referred to local centers for the important hands-on part— exercise, massage and acupuncture.

Considering mental activities, my most arduous mental task has been handling my own finances. Following Peter's death, I was faced with estate and income taxes in two countries, and the prospect of earning my own livelihood and supporting my growing son. My good attorney friend, Ruth, had helped me handle the estate issues. While Peter was alive, he handled the big financial decisions. Now with him gone, I needed to learn to manage these matters myself.

Six months after returning to Rochester, I bought a small house and started saving as much as I could from each pay check. When inflation soared in the 1980s, I was horrified to learn I was actually losing money by keeping it in the bank, since the interest earned on a saving account was less than the inflation rate. I was advised to buy stocks which would grow with inflation. Woefully ignorant on the subject, I turned to my father, who had stock experience and always had sound advice.

He said, "First, find a good stock broker—someone reliable who can help you. Start reading the papers and business magazines. Listen to the television programs about the economy and the stock market until you have a better understanding of the business world. Then, you can begin buying some stocks. Start with the bluest of the blue-chip companies, like General Electric, AT&T, Exxon." I followed his advice.

When I was working, I could only spend short periods on these matters. Now in retirement I began to maximize my assets to develop lifetime security. I carefully studied business newspapers and regularly listened to *Nightly Business Report* and *Wall Street Week with Louis Rukeyser*. With a trusted broker, I began to cautiously buy stocks and bonds with a portion of my savings. Investing, I discovered, was a combination of good information, good judgment and taking some risks. Since I am risk adverse, I chose conservative stocks and bonds of highest quality. I later located a sound financial advisor who showed me the wisdom of asset allocation—deciding what percentage of stocks, bonds and cash I should hold according to my risk tolerance and my lifetime horizon. He also encouraged me to diversify in each of these categories, such as growth stocks and value stocks, large cap and small cap stocks, treasury bonds and municipal bonds and so on. Adhering to these methods, I have built a solid underpinning for my future. I am convinced personal finance classes should be required in high school and college to help people learn wise financial management—a crucial part of survival. A secondary benefit from all this is it has made me a keen observer and follower of the economy, politics and world events.

I can see no way that these various mental stimuli—playing the piano, writing, advocating alternative therapies, managing finances and keeping up with the news—will diminish with time.

Next, I had to come to grips with some deep, troubling emotional issues that had too long lain dormant. The journey starts sadly but ends in happy triumph.

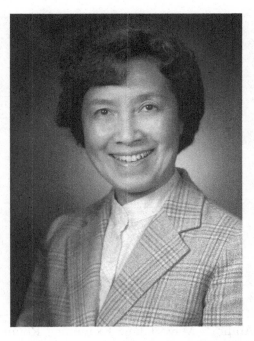

Author, Mayo Staff photo, 1985 (Mayo Photo Archives)

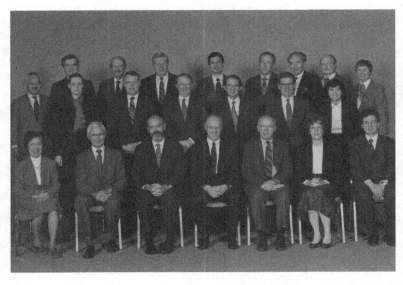

Mayo Rheumatology Division, 1990 (Mayo Photo Archives).

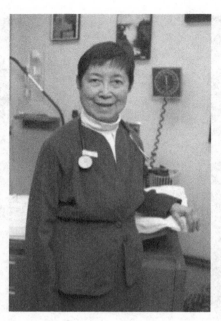

Author's Mayo Clinic Examining Room.

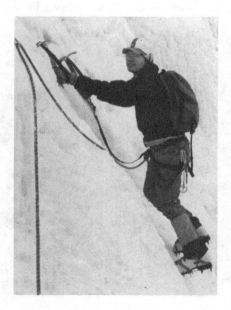

Son Paul Ice-climbing in Minnesota 1986

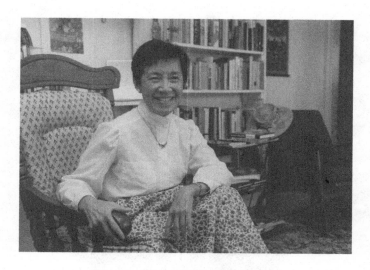

Author, retired, in Rochester home
(Photo permission from Rochester Post-Bulletin), 1992.

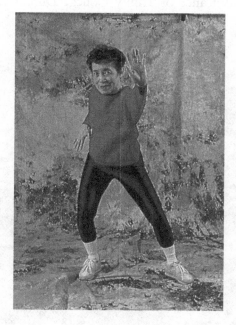

Author teaching Tai-chi, Mayo Fitness Center, 1997
(Mayo Photo Archives).

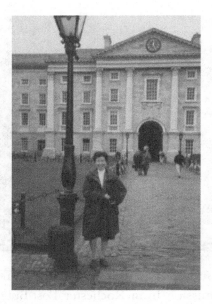

Author at Entrance of Trinity College Dublin University,
Dublin, Ireland, 1993.

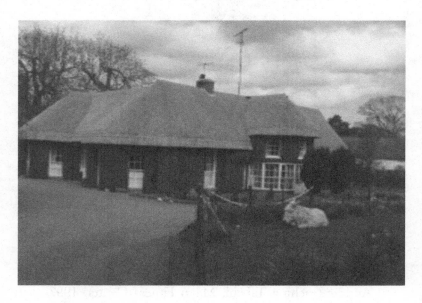

Thatched-roof cottage home of friends, Ireland 1993

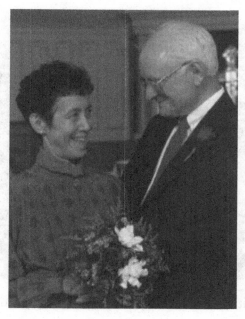

Wedding with Dr. Joseph C. Sharp, Rochester, MN 1996.

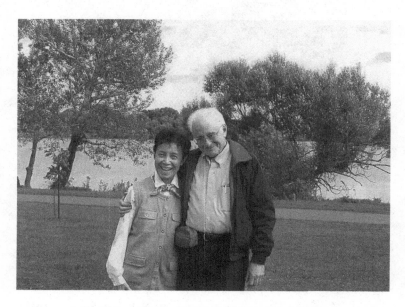

At Minneapolis Lake with husband Joe.

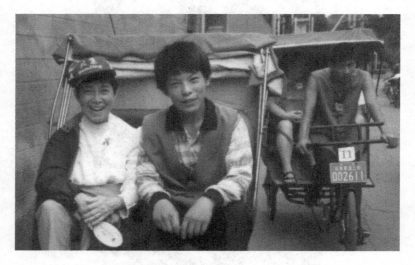

Author with pedicab driver, Beijing Hutong District, 1998.

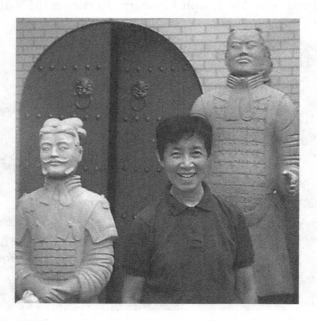

Author among terra cotta statues in Xi'an, China, 1998.

Chapter 15

RETIREMENT: EMOTIONAL PATHS,
PART I-IRELAND 1990-96

It was time to straighten out two troubling emotional issues. I dreaded and yet longed to start the healing process with final visits to both Ireland and China. It took a long time after Peter's death before I felt ready to return alone to Ireland, and even longer after my fearful escape to return to China.

On March 1993 my plane descended through the ever-present clouds over Dublin Airport, to see the familiar crazy quilt of small green and yellow fields, bordered by darker green hedges. Driving from the airport, I smelled the fresh earth and again felt the cold dampness on my cheek. After seventeen years, I was back in Ireland.

My friends, Elizabeth and John Kirker, whisked me to their home in Malahide, a northern suburb of Dublin. John, a neurologist, had been Peter's classmate in medical school, and Elizabeth my fondest friend in Ireland. Malahide's 1976 population of three thousand had burgeoned to eighteen thousand. New shops and houses filled the once empty areas in town and countryside. Ireland was reaping the rewards of increased commerce after joining the European Common Market (now the European Union).

I remembered their charming thatch-roofed cottage, set in a large green field where patches of yellow daffodils grew and a pair of white donkeys grazed. Although the Irish believed a thatched roof kept the house warm in winter and cool in summer, these houses have been rapidly disappearing. Elizabeth had remodeled the house interior into an elegant and comfortable home. A lovely slender blond, Elizabeth chatted cheerfully about her family, the house and the neighborhood, while I, in turn, brought her up to date about my family and work in Minnesota. After a supper featuring poached salmon with dill sauce, Irish brown soda bread and rhubarb fool we retired to the sitting room. There with humorous asides, John updated me on the changes in the local medical scene.

The next morning, sensing where my heart was, Elizabeth drove me to Peter's gravesite at St. Fintan's Cemetery in Sutton. To avoid the disheveled appearance of most Irish cemeteries, St. Fintan's had insisted on flat gravestones, flush with the ground, so the green grass around them could be mowed every week. The result was neat and orderly; the red and yellow tulips and daffodils hugging the stones gave a cheerful spring color. Peter's marble tablet was in a little curve of pink flowering shrubs. Its inscription, beautifully carved by his sculptress cousin, Hilary, stood out clearly. We wedged a water-filled glass jar of yellow daffodils, white virburnum and red japonica into the ground at the head of the stone. As I looked up at the mountains to the left, the sea to the right and the swooping gulls that filled the air with their cries, I thought, what a suitable resting place for my beloved Peter. Sitting there quietly reliving past times, I could almost hear Peter say, "Don't worry, my dear, it's alright." As his voice echoed in the wind, I suddenly felt a great peace.

That afternoon, my sister-in-law, Ann, picked me up to spend a few days on the south side of Dublin. I savored familiar scenes as the car sped along the coastal road from north to south of Dublin. In the early evening we arrived at Ann's comfortable little terrace house in Sandycove. An occupational therapist by profession, Ann had lived alone since my mother-in-law's death, but was now happily close to many friends and the school where she taught. I was comfortable with this wonderful, sensible woman.

We spent many hours discussing family, friends and conditions in Ireland. She told how Ireland's joining the European Union had initiated tremendous changes, giving them a new pride in being a nation whose opinion counted. With ease of travel to Europe, the Irish now looked toward the continent rather than inward at themselves. Foreign investments had poured in and the many factories built included American computer companies. These factories used the inexpensive local English-speaking work force to make goods to sell to the European continent. More employment and better wages gave the islanders a newfound sense of prosperity. For the first time, emigration slowed. Of course, as the standard of living rose, so did prices. Some prices for food and consumer goods even doubled. Sadly, drugs and serious crime had also been introduced. And the trouble with Northern Ireland remained unsettled, although the violence had abated.

From her place, I took the train into Dublin to visit the Psychiatry Department that Peter had established. Peter had his department headquarters at St. Patrick's Hospital and his dean's office at the Trinity College Dublin University campus. The Psychiatry Department had become a strong one. Professor Marcus Webb, a tall, graying, studious man, now its chairman, was full of welcome. I recalled the day Peter had proudly brought this promising young psychiatrist back from England to join his staff. We toured a new psychiatry building on the nearby St. James Hospital grounds, which had room for new buildings. I was excited to see how modern and well laid out the building was, and was especially pleased to see the two major wards named "Swift" and "Beckett"—honoring benefactors, Jonathan Swift, the writer and Peter Beckett, my husband. Marcus said, "The Psychiatry resident training program started by Peter continues strong and popular all over southern Ireland. Each year we also grant two Peter Beckett psychiatry awards to encourage young psychiatrists, just as he would have wished." I was happy and moved to see how successful Peter's last major efforts had become. His sacrifices seemed justified by these surviving legacies and warm memories. Marcus and I then walked a short way to St. Patrick's Hospital for lunch. Significantly, this has been Ireland's first psychiatric hospital, one of the oldest of its kind in the world. Jonathan Swift, its founder, had given his entire estate to it.

The following day, the retired chief of medicine, Dr. Gatenby, under whom I had worked, invited me to tour the campus grounds of Trinity College University Dublin. The Dean's office was much as I remembered—a comfortable wood-paneled room with a large wooden desk and walls lined with book-filled shelves. Dr. Gatenby said last year he had helped host several hundred medical alumni who came from all over the world to celebrate Trinity's 400th anniversary. He had been busy taking them around the university grounds as he was doing with me. We lunched in a building called Commons. Looking back, I vividly recall attending an important dinner in its great dining hall. I had viewed with awe the walls that were lined with huge portraits of past provosts and dignitaries, and the gleaming silverware on the long U-shaped table. We were dressed in our finery, the men in tuxedos and the women in long formal gowns. Students in dark suits waited on tables, a young woman played the harp and prayers were intoned in Latin. When I praised the pomp and splendor of the occasion, my table companion growled, "These traditions are chains, chains to the past," an interesting viewpoint.

We were now served lunch cafeteria-style in an adjacent smaller room, where I met several old faculty friends. Afterward, as was customary, we went upstairs to drink coffee in the lounge, where the professors chatted and read the daily papers. One jokingly said to me, "This place is ruined now that we allow women in." Were they still uneasy at the presence of women, I wondered?

Dr. Gatenby then walked me through an attractive new bookstore into the famous Trinity Library. Scholars came from all over the world to study in the Library's enormous collection of distinguished old books. On a wooden pedestal in one corner lay the Book of Kells, a beautiful Bible considered the finest example of medieval monastic art. It was opened to show a hand-illustrated page of ornate writing in gold, red and blue ink. As I walked along, I photographed both the inside and outside of those lovely old university buildings with their rich past. In retrospect, during the crowded day, I did not have opportunity to ask what changes in thoughts and conditions had taken place among faculty and students. I did remember being told Catholic students were no longer banned from attending this Protestant Trinity College.

Ann and I spent the next two days visiting favorite old haunts. Buttoning up our anoraks against the cold wind, we walked along the sea. Gray mists filled the cloudless skies, and cold wet spray stung our faces. We stopped at the home office of Eoin O'Brien, the Irish editor of many Samuel Beckett's literary works. After introductions, he sold me a copy of his new book *The Beckett Country, Samuel Beckett's Ireland*, not yet available in America. This handsomely illustrated book describes Sam's Irish origins and the source of many scenes in his plays. What a coup to have my own precious record of the Beckett family background shared by Peter and Sam.

On another day, Ann and I drove through the Wicklow Mountains, south of Dublin. The Beckett family had loved spending weekends driving, climbing and picnicking among these treeless, bog-soaked hills. I too learned to love these drives. We saw familiar turf diggers scoop up the compressed vegetation with brick-shaped turf spades. They cut turf, piled them up in cones to dry, and later transported them down as fuel to warm homes. When looking at these hills from afar, in a certain light they appeared dark blue, as in the paintings of well-known artist Jack Yeats. Later in spring, Ann said, they turned yellow when the tiny yellow flowers of the ubiquitous gorse shrub emerged.

In the lower levels of the hills, we passed small villages and many old ruins of stone buildings that lay amid the nettles and grasses. In a graveyard, adjacent to an ancient little church, we found moss-encrusted tombstones inscribed with barely decipherable dates of two to three hundred years ago. Scattered between the tombstones stood ancient Celtic crosses (a circle in the middle of the cross). Nearby, a flock of sheep grazed on a hilly slope. A shepherd whistled sharp commands to his dog, and we saw the dog running and barking to herd the sheep.

We found the Avoca wool shop in a dip in the hills. This cottage industry was known for exquisite gossamer wool of unusual blends of color. We watched a weaver working at his loom, and bought two scarves: a blend of dusky pink and white for Ann, and one of blue and mauve for me. Every site and edifice had a story, real or fancied, all dear to the Irish heart.

The last day of my visit ended in a light-hearted party given by John and Elizabeth in their home. Physicians, businessmen and politicians brought their wives to a sumptuous meal with free-flowing wine and conversation. Glasses were raised to friendships and reunions. I expressed hope their European liaison would bring ever larger vision and more prosperity to this small green island at the edge of the Atlantic Ocean.

I was glad to have returned. Peter had dearly loved his native country. The peace I felt at his grave, and the warm welcome of my friends and family finally brought closure to my Irish experience. The unique charm of this land and its people will always tug at my heart.

A wonderful thing happened after I got back to Minnesota. I belonged to a Macintosh computer users group of congenial Clinic colleagues. One day, Dr. Joe Sharp from the Medical Science division, came to speak about "computer viruses." I learned a computer virus was not a biological organism, but was as aggressive and destructive as a living virus. When I asked him for more details, he offered to come to my house to check my computer for viruses, and to add a program to protect it from future intrusions. Shortly afterward, he attended a Pritikin health workshop in California, and returned to convert me to a new way of cooking and eating, volunteering to be my official taster. From there our friendship grew. Of medium build, a head taller than I, glasses and clean-shaven, he reminded me of a cheerful, friendly mischievous gnome, full of enthusiasm and ideas—a free spirit. A month after meeting him, I scrawled this description.

> Who is Joe, who is he?
> Twinkling eyes, and gentle heart.
> A shock of white hair,
> A razor keen mind,
> That is Joe,
> My newfound friend.

He knows wonder,
He loves beauty.
He likes people.
He helps others,
That is Joe,
My newfound friend.

We both liked music, he especially Baroque, so we went to concerts together. We found we enjoyed many things in common in addition to music—food, books and an endless interest in new ideas. Meals became prolonged discussions. Although he soon finished his stint at Mayo and moved to Minneapolis, we kept in touch by extensive e-mail. On a bright, warm sunny day in September 1996, our friendship culminated in a simple family wedding in my church chapel. The wedding party consisted of our immediate family members and a few close friends. I wore a turquoise silk dress with a deep pink neck scarf and Joe was resplendent in a black suit with a red tie. In the reception in my home afterward, we feasted on delicious Chinese dishes from our favorite Chinese restaurant, and a carrot wedding cake. It was a glorious occasion.

We found marriage between two mature professionals quite unlike that of two young people starting out. We each had definite ideas, strong opinions and settled ways. But we quickly learned to tolerate each other's idiosyncrasies, to agree to disagree on certain matters and above all to strengthen our mutual bonds. We admired each other's strengths and tried to help each other in our weaknesses. To our dismay, we had the nuisance of eliminating duplicate books, computers, furniture and unfortunately, junk—both of us being accumulators. Happily, we remain optimists and futurists, sharing the joy of living in a time of exciting changes and discoveries.

To find a wonderful companion at this late stage of life was beyond anything I could have imagined. How fortunate for me! Now, together, we can explore further adventures.

Chapter 16

RETIREMENT:

EMOTIONAL PATHS, PART II-CHINA 1996-

2000

Soon after our marriage, Joe and I began discussing a trip to China. I had long wanted to go, but was apprehensive about going alone. Joe felt China was becoming a great power and wanted to see the country of my birth.

I had strong mixed feelings about going. During the fifty years since I fled the Sino-Japanese war, China had undergone tumultuous changes. The ten-year Japanese war had beggared the nation and killed millions, including half of my extended family. Mao Zedong, the leader of the Chinese Communists, took control of China in 1949. At first a revolutionary, he later became a tyrant. He jailed or killed whole classes of people—landowners, business people and academics—who threatened his absolute authority, including many members of my father's family. Millions also died in famines and political upheavals. These actions bitterly alienated me. However, to his credit, Mao unified the country by creating a strong central government, built roads linking cities and established Mandarin as the single official dialect. Over time, he improved the people's food and housing, reduced illiteracy, established a medical system that stopped epidemics, and put the nation on a bumpy course toward economic progress.

In 1972 President Nixon reopened communications between China and America. After Mao's death in 1976, the next leader, Deng Xiaoping, introduced a market economy by loosening the government's stranglehold on entrepreneurs and trade. Jiang Zemin, who followed him, further enlarged this policy. As the country's economic health steadily improved, the government control lessened. Watching from afar, I began to hope China would rejoin the international community of nations. Because my father had been an official of the rival Nationalist Government, I was afraid the Chinese authorities might arbitrarily detain me, so I felt much safer accompanied by Joe, an outspoken, bonafide American citizen. We decided to tour two cities, Beijing and Xi'an, in a ten day period. We were eager to see first-hand how new developments affected the lives of the people.

We arrived at Beijing airport on a hot, sticky late June afternoon in 1998. After an hour of good-natured confusion, Kung, our tour guide, found us and brought us to a modern five-star hotel, which provided luxurious comfort. Beijing, present capital of China in Hebei Province[18], is about a hundred miles inland from the China Sea on the northeastern coast. Its population was twelve million. Our tour started with visits to ancient buildings and historic sites.

On the first morning, Kung guided us through the Forbidden City, residence of past emperors, where the general population had been forbidden to enter. The imperial palace grounds in

---

[18] Province: an administrative division of China. They are larger than our states; their boundaries often follow natural geographic lines.

central Beijing still awe visitors. Built during the previous Ming dynasty[19], 1368-1644, its rectangular shape is half a mile from east to west, two-thirds of a mile from north to south, surrounded by a high wall and a deep moat. The imperial complex is arranged along a central north-south axis, which is entered through a series of gates from the south entrance. The emperor held ceremonies and conducted business in the "outer court," the southern front half; the royal family lived in the "inner court," the northern back half of the complex. The whole area consists of many small houses, each with its own courtyard. The priceless treasures that once filled the nine thousand rooms have since been moved to national museums. These wooden houses, brightly painted vermilion and green, stand on white marble terraces, their gold-tiled conical roofs glittering in the sun. The emperor with his family and retinue had lived here in lavish luxury, isolated from the common people.

On our second morning, we visited the site of the Ming Tombs northwest of Beijing, where thirteen Ming emperors had been buried at the foot of the Tianshou Mountains. We walked along a stone path, the Sacred Way, flanked on both sides by handsome twelve-foot tall stone statues of warriors, officials and animals such as lions, camels, elephants and horses. We smilingly posed for each other's snapshots standing beside the statues. At the end of the path a museum exhibited rare and beautiful objects in gold, silver, pearl, jade and porcelain, which had been stored in an emperor's tomb.

In the afternoon, we climbed the renowned Great Wall. Kung told us its construction began when China first became a nation during the Qin dynasty, about 220 BCE. Starting just

---

[19] Dynasty: a succession of rulers who are members of the same family or group. China's history is dated by a sequence of dynasties, each with their distinctive names.

north of Xi'an in central China, subsequent dynasties had gradually extended the wall eastward. It twists through mountains and grasslands like a giant serpent for nearly two thousand miles until it reaches the sea, just north of Beijing. It is the only man-made structure visible to our astronauts in space. I shuddered at the thought of the millions of forced laborers that died in its building. Although intended to prevent invasions by northern nomadic steppe people, these same people penetrated it twice to conquer China. We ascended the hill by cable car to the base of the wall, then walked up a long stairway to the top for a spectacular view of the surrounding mountains. I rested and took pictures, while others walked along the wall.

What had I seen of the people during these days?

The huge number of people on bicycles stunned me. They streamed in two to three irregular columns on both sides of the main street, leaving the center four lanes for auto traffic. I was surprised everyone dressed in Western rather than the traditional Chinese clothes. The clean-shaven men with close-cropped hair, wore open collar short-sleeve shirts and long dark pants. The women with boyish haircuts or longer hair tied neatly in back with a ribbon, wore colorful blouses or tunics and dark slacks. Everyone appeared healthy and lean. I saw few children or white-haired folks and was told the children were in school and the elderly at home. I heard friendly talk and laughter, and found the people on the street courteously helpful to us tourists.

Well-stocked small shops lined the central Beijing streets, selling food, clothes and household objects. People darted in and out of them, purchases in hand. Bold skyscraper hotels and office buildings loomed along the main streets, marked with both Chinese and English signs—Beijing Hotel, Siemens, Hewlett-Packard, McDonalds. Unfortunately, a haze of air pollution covered the city, containing (we were told) a mixture of burning coal fumes, car exhaust and widespread cigarette smoke. I developed an irritating cough that persisted for many days after returning to America.

The currency exchange, Kung said, was 8.27 yuan to an U.S. dollar. The average per capita income, equivalent to two thousand dollars a year, made it impossible for individuals to buy a home or car, a new privilege granted by the government. Most people lived in subsidized rented apartments, and traveled by foot, bicycle, bus or train. Still, the people seemed to feel they were much better off in recent years.

With pride, Kung told us education was free, even though children and adults were tested at every level before advancing. Should they fail, they had to leave school to find less desirable work, so the push for education was intense. Although there were a number of famous Beijing universities, we were unable to gain entrance without knowing someone inside.

Health care, Kung said, was also free, but difficult to obtain. Except for a few outstanding hospitals in Beijing, medical care for the bulk of the population was probably mediocre. Most people first went to eastern herbal doctors, and only if not cured sought help from western-trained medical doctors. Kung managed to get us into the Eastern Medicine Center in Beijing, where I learned to do deep therapeutic massage on my husband's chronic stiff neck. "It's the best thing you learned on the trip," Joe joked.

Our hotel provided bountiful breakfast buffets and several excellent restaurants. Tap water was not safe, so we drank bottled water, bottled soft drinks, boiled water, hot tea or coffee. Alcoholic drinks were easily available. I explained to my husband that since North China produced wheat, the standard dishes were steamed buns, often with delicious meat stuffing, and noodles, rather than his favorite rice, a warm weather crop of the South. Tasty, but rich roast Peking duck was a local specialty.

We had a rare opportunity to contrast living conditions in Beijing at two different levels. Kung secured an optional trip for eight of us to visit the Beijing *hutongs*, the city's poor district. Adjacent to the Forbidden City, this area was once a luxurious living place for high nobles and visiting dignitaries. When the Qing dynasty fell in 1911, the area went into decline and the poor moved in. We were told about three million people lived there. *Hutong* stands for the narrow lanes connecting the many small houses. Too narrow for cars, entrance into the area could only be by walking, bicycling or *pedicab* (a three-wheeled two-seater bicycle peddled by a young man). The friendly pedicab man, who brought us, said he wanted to come to America. Our group crowded into the home of a middle-aged woman and her adult son. She welcomed us with a smile, and fed us watermelon as we sat on her chairs and bed, asking questions through our interpreter guide. She showed us her four small rooms: two bedrooms, a living room and a kitchen. She cooked with coal fire, had electricity and running water and used a public bathroom down the alley. We saw a small refrigerator, two tiny television sets and a bicycle by the door. She appeared to be enormously pleased with her lot. We were impressed that living conditions, even in the poor district, were reasonably adequate.

The living condition of our Chinese professional contact was quite different. He had lived in the U.S. and now worked for IBM in Beijing to help the eager Chinese learn and use computers. His work place was in the Lido Hotel complex, which not only contained a modern hotel with conference rooms, but was also linked to offices with computers and an elegant self-contained shopping mall. After showing us around, he graciously invited us to supper in his attractive two-story house in a gated park. The house had every modern convenience, including a maid and cook. We had a delightful evening with his family, in what could have been in the home of an American businessman.

On another free afternoon we visited a Chinese businessman from Minneapolis who managed Honeywell's office for North China. His family lived in an apartment in the diplomatic zone in central Beijing. During lunch, he described how his Chinese background and sensitivity to local conditions helped him persuade several Chinese firms to buy the Honeywell thermostatic control system. After lunch, he walked us to two of Beijing's best bookstores, crammed with books and crowded with young buyers. The Chinese books were almost all in paperback and very cheap. My husband exclaimed in amazement, "Look at this computer book that's just been published in the U.S. It's already translated into Chinese. The price is half what it is at home." I bought an illustrated Tai-chi exercise book to use for my class. Joe and I felt convinced these bilingual, bicultural Chinese, educated and trained in the U.S., will have enormous influence on China's move into the modern world.

After four days in Beijing, we flew in a 737 China Airlines plane to Xi'an. This city is about five hundred fifty miles southwest of Beijing, in the province of Shaanxi, with six million inhabitants. Bao-li, our local guide, said dating from 220 BCE, this was the capital of the powerful First Emperor, who vanquished then united rival ethnic states to establish the first Chinese dynasty, named Qin. From here the Great Wall stretched toward the east, and the famous Silk Road stretched toward the west. The latter was China's only contact with the West for centuries. Many subsequent dynasties had their capitals here, the last one being the great Tang dynasty, about 600-900 CE, which the local people still celebrate in festivals. We liked this spacious, less crowded city with purer air than Beijing.

We had all come to see the recently unearthed terra cotta army, built and buried by the First Emperor to protect him in his after life. Housed in an enormous cavern excavated in the 1980s, this six-to-eight thousand-man army could be viewed by visitors, even as excavations continued. This archeological find of the century made Xi'an an outstanding tourist attraction. The slightly taller than life figures, made of local terra cotta clay, had been sculpted, fired at 1000 degrees Fahrenheit for a week, then glazed and painted. Each life-like face had a distinctive individual shape and expression, no doubt representing a specific soldier. They were magnificent, even though their original brilliant colors had faded in the two thousand years the figures had lain there. Visitors were not allowed to take pictures of the warriors, but we could view them from a balcony above. We were amused to see a special staircase being built for President Clinton's later visit, so he could descend and stand alongside these figures. We jokingly told everyone we were part of Clinton's advance team.

At my husband's special request, we visited the Forest of Steles. This unusual museum of stone tablets, many ten feet tall, displayed examples of the finest Chinese calligraphy (a distinctive art form of writing) carved and preserved in stone. The seventeen hundred tablets in these pavilions captured the changing writing styles over this long period dating from the Han dynasty (about 200 BCE-200 CE) until recent years. Confucian classics were the major subject of the tablet writings. Since antiquity, scholars have come to view and study these remarkable tablets. I bought two rubbings of a style of writing to practice calligraphy at home.

My husband told me about two striking places on the tour, which I missed because of my tired legs and swollen feet. One was a live animal market, where to his astonishment, vendors were busy peddling noisy dogs, goats, pigs, snakes, fish, pheasants and other creatures destined for the cooking pots. The other was the Shaanxi Provincial Historical Museum containing archaeological finds portraying over five thousand years of human civilization. There were all types of relics, including those of bone, wood, early metals and precious stones. This city is truly an archeologist's paradise.

Our two excellent tour guides became our most intimate contacts with local Chinese. Both men worked for the China International Travel Service, a government agency managing nearly all foreign visits. After a college degree, they trained another two years to study the specific language and culture of a country they would specialize in. Both men worked hard to balance accurate information about toured places with truthful answers to our many questions.

Kung, our Beijing guide, was a serious young man of about thirty-five, wearing a T-shirt emblazoned with "Hard Rock" printed on the front, and "Save the Lonely Planet" on the back, long dark pants and leather walking shoes. He carried a cell phone that was in continuous use as he arranged activities for our tour. It seemed everyone carried cell phones, since the lack of built-in phones lines left this as the only practical way of communication. He was prompt, efficient and spoke English with only a slight accent. To my husband's question on freedom of speech, he answered, "We don't have freedom of speech yet, but we do have opportunities for courage." When asked why we saw so few signs indicating gas stations on the road, he replied, "Reform in the past ten years has brought many changes. Gas stations had been placed where only government officials could find them, but they are slowly putting up signs for ordinary drivers."

Kung wondered aloud why Americans insisted on "human rights" in China. He felt recent reforms had greatly improved the lot of ordinary people. They had food, shelter, jobs, free education and medical care, and recently, freedom to buy housing and to travel in China. He thought they already achieved human rights. We then realized these two words had a different meaning for us and for many Chinese.

Bao-li, our Xi'an guide was an entirely different personality. A little older, he had combed-back hair, and a broad handsome face, which was seldom without a smile. His English was slow and precise, and he liked to joke. He was proud of his city, and was anxious we see as much of its culture and history as we could fit in; he happily arranged the special trips to show us glimpses of life in Xi'an. Like many parents there, Bao-li was anxiously awaiting results of his young son's high school examination. He and his son showed great interest when my husband talked about computers for communication and information. "Next time you hear from me, it will be by e-mail," Bao-li promised with a big laugh. We liked both men; we believe such bright, ambitious and resourceful people will thrive in the new China.

I left China with a buoyant feeling of hope and pride. After great upheavals, the people and nation have emerged stronger. The nation is dynamic and on the move, and the people see better things ahead. Even if I never visit China again, I will always be proud of my heritage.

I want to emphasize how much deeper my friendships became during my retirement. Now that I had time I went on a flurry of trips to visit family and friends. I dropped in several times on my sister in New York, and my brother in Cleveland. I spent time with old friends in Detroit, and Grand Rapids. My friends and I took trips together, to Disney World in Orlando, to the Bahamas, to Maine, to Palm Beach, to New Orleans, on ships on the Mississippi, and on larger ships in Alaska. I joined friends on Elderhostel trips to S. Carolina, and the Twin Cities, and sat rapt listening to plays at the Shakespeare Festival in

Canada. It was exciting to be with friends on oversea tours to Greece & Italy, Denmark & Sweden, and even to exotic Thailand, Singapore & Hongkong. I made several trips to see La Dunn in her hide-out in the N. Carolina mountains. In Minnesota, I drove to spend time with friends in Duluth and New Ulm. Everywhere I also made new friends. I simply had a wonderful time talking, eating and sharing with these precious people who enriched my life.

I have come full circle bringing closure to hurtful experiences in Ireland and China; I have made my peace with each of them. Friends, family and a new life companion offer a springboard to future happiness. My spiritual quest is the next thing to explore, the nebulous, mysterious journey we must all make sooner or later.

Chapter 17

RETIREMENT:

SPIRITUAL PATHS 1990-2000

My most difficult, yet rewarding retirement activity has been a spiritual search. I wanted to confront several issues in exploring my paths to God and to life. How could I reconcile the inexplicable deaths of husband and son? What really was my Christian faith? What spiritual path could I follow in this new millennium? Since my personality, cultural background and experiences play a strong part in what is right for me, the result might not hold for anyone else. I discovered this when Joe and I found we agreed on some issues, but differed on others.

Born in China of an agnostic father and a Christian mother, she made sure I was baptized and attended Sunday school. The American Protestant missionaries who frequented my home brought Christian sayings and hymns into my daily life. I had attended Christian schools, received medical care in Christian hospitals and Christian missionaries were instrumental in my coming to America. "Fellowship" meant helping each other in the Christian family.

Even though I came to America as a young foreign woman, on my own with limited funds, I felt secure because of my membership in the Christian church. It offered access to a national community of kind people whom I trusted to help me if I was in need. Later as an adult, the church has been my Sunday morning haven where I could worship, sing and unwind from a stressful week. Its pervasive goodness covered me like a warm protective blanket, which I accepted without much thought about the basic tenets of faith.

The early death of my first husband shattered this complacent faith. All that felt firm and dependable in my life collapsed. After the initial shock and tears, I became angry with God who I felt punished us unfairly. I also was disappointed in my church for not answering my question "Why?" Since I had urgent practical matters to attend then, I hid this jumble of pain in a corner of my consciousness.

Two decades later, a Rochester support group unexpectedly helped me unleash a torrent of long-buried emotions to leave me finally feeling released and cleansed. When I later studied psychology, I learned powerful feelings had to be faced before they could be resolved. Not only must I talk things out, I had to think my way through them. This need became more pressing when my only son died suddenly.

After a long search of religious and secular literature, I found an answer in Rabbi Harold Kushner's 1981 book *When Bad Things Happen to Good People*. He came to terms with the death of his teenage son after studying the book of Job in the Old Testament. Kushner reasoned God made human life to follow natural physiological laws, such as birth, illness, maturity, aging, etc. Then He gave man free will, to choose and bear the consequences of his own choices. Pursuing this logic, I came to believe that Kushner's son, and my husband and son had succumbed to basic forces. No one was to blame. God would not tamper with His own laws. Nevertheless, He feels our pain, and is there to sustain us in our suffering with His great love and support. Thinking this way, I could finally put away my sadness and hurt, freeing me to dwell on memories of our happy times together.

One wintry day, as I sat near a sunny window in my living room, my thoughts turned to my son, Paul. On a table by my side was a small tray of polished stones and shells, a potted green fern and two tiny figurines—all gifts from him. Even as a child of three Paul loved stones, I was afraid he would swallow those he carried in his mouth. At eight, his pants pockets had holes from jammed-in stones. As a teenager, he collected and polished unusual stones, tagging them to show where he found them. The stones he gave me were one-to-two inches long, shiny and smooth, purple, red, or green, seamed with wavy lines. I liked to rub my fingers over them.

Paul and I shared a passion for collecting shells and sea fossils. They came from lakes in Michigan, the seashore in Maui, Hawaii, the Jamaican coast on the Caribbean, the cliff walk in Ireland, Lake Superior near Duluth University and the beach of his favorite park south of Berkeley, California. Our favorites were the long or round spiral shells, the rough oyster shell, the starfish, the sand dollar and the fan-shaped scallop shell. The small ones on the tray reminded me of the lovely days wandering together at the water's edge.

My glance then fell on the small pot of filmy-leafed green fern. Ten years prior, Paul had hand-carried it from Duluth, Minnesota, to give me something in the house to enjoy during the long winter. When I watered it each week, I felt I was saying hello to him. He had absorbed his father's love of the outdoors, finding joy in parks and water shores. Camping, hiking and rock climbing became essential parts of his life, and seemed to renew his spirit.

He also attended ceramic workshops, sending me vases and platters that had beauty and vitality. His art seemed to capture strong feelings he found hard to express in words. Two tiny figurines on the table, a Buddha and a turtle, were the last things he sent me. The Buddha, about an inch-and-a-half tall, of a dark gray surface with silver tones, had a wide smile on his face. The little turtle, of the same length, had a smooth, light green outer shell. According to Chinese legend, the laughing Buddha is the symbol of happiness, and the turtle a symbol of long life—Paul's last wishes for me. I realized for the first time that Peter and Paul live on in me because they are alive in my head—Peter that wonderful, solid man and Paul the gentle, loving soul. It is their essence and smiling presence I will always remember.

After clarifying my feelings toward God and becoming reconciled to my bereavement, I began to question what constituted my Christian faith. I came upon *Mere Christianity* by C. S. Lewis, 1943, an English writer on moral issues. Initially a non-believer, he described how he came to believe in Christianity. His clear, logical thought and inspired reasoning helped me understand the basic tenets of my religion.

Just as I naively believed I understood Christianity, I was shaken to read *The Gospel According to Jesus* published in 1991 by the biblical scholar Stephen Mitchell. It gave me a different slant. Like Thomas Jefferson, he selected those parts of the Four Gospels he felt to be the authentic Jesus, and rejected the confused and contradictory parts he thought had been added by later authors. Jesus emerged as a remarkable teacher of exceptional spirituality, who preached love and forgiveness in a world torn by hate and violence. He used simple, powerful stories to teach us to love God with all our hearts and our neighbor as ourselves. The stories of the Good Samaritan and the woman to be stoned particularly moved me.

The first told of a man lying wounded on the ground after bandits stole his goods and beat him. Passersby ignored him until a Samaritan, a man from an ethnic group considered enemies by his people, stopped to take care of him. The lesson shows us compassion has no boundaries. In the other, seeing a woman accused of adultery and about to be stoned by a crowd, Jesus said, "Let you who have no sin, throw the first stone." The crowd slunk away. Since we are all prone to mistakes and wrong doings, this story teaches us to show others the same mercy and forgiveness we wish to receive. After Jesus died a martyr, his disciples widely disseminated his teachings to develop Christianity as a formalized religion. Later the church fathers added dogmas and rituals, and proclaimed new beliefs— some I found hard to accept. The original pristine teachings and enduring love of Jesus remain the core of my beliefs.

As the year 2000 arrived, I asked my pastor, "What message is emerging from the best minds of our Protestant churches to inspire and invigorate us in this new millennium? Surely the teachings of two thousand years ago need to be reviewed and reinterpreted in the light of today's world." The graying of my church congregation dramatizes our need to invigorate our church by attracting young families. How can we reach this younger generation? And how can I adapt my own beliefs to the present?

As technology and economics begin to dominate our country, the traditional religious institutions no longer seem relevant to many young people, who are actively exploring non-mainstream beliefs. A young Catholic friend ignores her church's stand on divorce and contraception. A cousin attends a group that believes in the special power of Light. National boundaries and ethnicity fade as people move easily between countries. Patients come to the Mayo Clinic from countries with no prior presence here. At my local supermarket, I hear languages from Asia, Africa, Middle East and Latin America.

Our school children from these different backgrounds are easily learning to mix cultures. The European Union further unified Western Europe by launching the euro and issuing a common passport. A friend said, "A girl in Norway can have boyfriends in France, Holland and Italy." We are becoming one world at an accelerating pace.

To add to this change and confusion, the headlines scream of bomb threats, ethnic cleansing, drug trafficking, terrorism, gun violence and religious strife. I ask, "How are today's leaders in churches, synagogues, mosques and temples guiding our spiritual growth and promoting social harmony?

Hearing no clear reply, I began exploring various religious practices at home and abroad myself. In the 1980s I had toured lands of ancient religions. I had walked where Jesus trod in Jerusalem and Galilee; knelt without shoes in the golden-domed Great Mosque of Jerusalem, sacred to Muslims; listened to the Pope in Rome; and lit a temple candle before a Buddhist priest in Thailand. Much as I valued these experiences, I gained no new insights.

In Rochester, I spent a week's retreat in a Catholic motherhouse, where I slept in a bare room with only a bed, desk and a cross on the wall, and passed the day in prayer and lectures. I had felt God's presence in a Unitarian church and a Quaker meeting. The Greek Orthodox Church took me back to Byzantine times with its icons, incense and cantor singing. An ecumenical Thanksgiving service in our local synagogue was much like one in my own church, except for the brief showing of the Torah. I still had not found my pathway. I asked myself, in what practical ways could I fulfill God's wish and my spiritual life? Unlike some admirable friends, I am not a volunteer by nature; I have no inclination to rush off to Africa to feed hungry children, nor to devote time in my community to doing "good works."

My epiphany came from two books and a recent Minneapolis talk by the Dalai Lama. He profoundly altered my outlook. He is the exiled spiritual and temporal leader of the Buddhist Tibetan people and the winner of the 1989 Nobel Peace Prize. The books detailing his views are *The Art of Happiness* 1998 (authored by American psychiatrist Dr. Howard C. Cutler) and *The Ethics for the New Millennium* 1999.

In *The Art of Happiness* Dr. Cutler interviews the Dalai Lama to identify principles that guide this intelligent, inspiring man to be serene in spite of his adversities. The Dalai Lama begins with the observation that we are all fellow human beings who want to be happy and avoid suffering. He believes we can each achieve happiness by training our mind and heart, thereby transforming our attitude toward life. He calls his training "inner discipline." We must identify our negative thoughts, feelings and behavior so we can gradually eliminate them, and uncover our positive thoughts, feelings and behavior so we can cultivate and enhance them. Negative traits (qualities that hurt others), include anger, envy, hatred, violence, greed, etc. Positive traits (qualities that help others), include compassion, tolerance, forgiveness, humility, generosity, etc. In short, he asks us to first examine our lives, then methodically change it for the better. One person might find he is envious but kind, while another is violent but honest. Each must work on ridding negative traits and strengthening positive ones.

Paradoxically, as we help others be happier, the Dalai Lama says, we become happier ourselves. Furthermore, he tells us, this training begets a calmness and peace of mind that buffers us against suffering and difficulties that come to us all. Although simple in theory this valuable training is difficult to achieve, so he recommends a lifetime of daily thought and meditation. I came to realize that this is a specific personal path to change by one's own efforts (Buddhists do not believe in an external God, although there is a sense of a Godhead).

When searching the subject of meditation, I found most help from *The New Three Minute Meditator* 1990, by David Harp with Nina Feldman. After a halting start, I began to teach it to my Tai-chi Yoga class. Toward the end of the class hour, as the students lay supine on their mats, I turned up the slow music in the background. Then I instructed them to close their eyes and slowly relax. "Relax your feet. Relax your calves. Relax your pelvis. Relax your back . . . ." and so on up the body to, "Relax your eyes. Relax your jaws." Next, I asked them to, "Clear your mind of all distracting thoughts. Tell them to go away, you'll deal with them later. Just concentrate on your breathing, Inhale . . . Out, Inhale . . . Out. Let the music sweep through your body. You'll stay like this three minutes." After three minutes, I asked them to stand up and take the Sun Salute pose (full body stretch) to end the class. As Î guided the weekly class, I really learned the three-minute, mind-clearing meditation, and it became a big help in stressful times. Although a simplified form of meditation, it proved a fruitful beginning.

Attempting the "inner discipline" was even more challenging. Although usually patient, I could swiftly become angry if someone pushes a vulnerable button. One day Joe came to the supper table after a tiring day. The dish I had cooked turned out badly and I was fuming when we sat down. "I'm hot," I snapped. "Why didn't you come to the table when I called?" He replied in irritation, "Stop complaining, or I'll leave the table." I retorted, "This is my house and I'll complain if I want to." He left the table and went to his study. Alone and shaking with fury I could not eat; I just sat there until I finally simmered down. Pause . . . I thought, this anger is ridiculous . . . it does neither of us any good. Pause . . . . It's over such a trivial matter . . . . frustration with my cooking.

Then I remembered how unpleasant it was for Joe when his mother carped at him at the table. Ruefully, I missed our usual laughing table conversations. Recalling how caring he was when I was ill, my anger promptly evaporated. A hard lesson—be more patient and avoid anger. And this was just one of my negative traits! This was going to be a long, slow process, but I comforted myself with the thought, it's the journey that matters, more than the destination.

In *Ethics for the New Millennium* the Dalai Lama broadens his basic concept. To the poor in backward countries who suffer from want and misery (outward suffering), and to the rich in developed countries who suffer from anxiety and depression (inward suffering), he proposes a personal "spiritual revolution" his "inner discipline" as the solution. Anyone can practice this discipline irrespective of religion, age, race or culture.

The Dalai Lama also wants us to extend our self-improvement to others in our society, not by proselytizing, but by example. He believes our inner discipline and peace will gradually ripple throughout our world. He also believes a variety of religions should coexist in harmony, since people have different personalities and come from diverse cultures and beliefs. I am in complete agreement, for this kind of diversity makes the world more challenging and interesting. After all, my background mingles several cultures.

These teachings touch a deep cord within me. They crystallize much of what I have experienced and believe. I can practice this inner discipline by thought and meditation in the quiet of my own home. My spiritual path in the new millennium is clear. I want to follow Jesus' teachings, practice this discipline, while I respect others who follow their own spiritual road map.

I have opened many new doors in retirement. For continued physical health, I will diet and exercise; for mental health, I will keep up with events in science, economics and politics; for emotional health, I will maintain close contacts with friends and family; and for spiritual health I will practice this discipline.

"What next?" Joe asks. I eagerly reply, "I'm sure more doors will open. Who knows what surprising new joys are around the corner.